AYURVEDA FOR BEGINNERS:
Ayurvedic practices for natural healing

WARREN DYLOG

Copyright © 2020 **Warren Dylog**

All rights reserved.
This document is geared towards providing exact and reliable information with regards to the topic and issue covered. The publication is sold with the idea that the publisher is not required to render accounting, officially permitted, or otherwise, qualified services. If advice is necessary, legal or professional, a practiced individual in the profession should be ordered.

-From a Declaration of Principles which was accepted and approved equally by a Committee of the American Bar Association and a Commit
tee of Publishers and Associations.

In no way is it legal to reproduce, duplicate, or transmit any part of this document in either electronic means or in printed format. Recording of this publication is strictly prohibited and any storage of this document is not allowed unless with written permission from the publisher.All rights reserved.

The information provided herein is stated to be truthful and consistent, in that any liability, in terms of inattention or otherwise, by any usage or abuse of any policies, processes, or directions contained within is the solitary and utter responsibility of the recipient reader. Under no circumstances will any legal responsibility or blame be held against the publisher for any reparation, damages, or monetary loss due to the information herein, either directly or indirectly.

Respective authors own all copyrights not held by the publisher.

The information herein is offered for informational purposes solely, and is universal as so. The presentation of the information is without contract or any type of guarantee assurance.
The trademarks that are used are without any consent, and the publication of the trademark is without permission or backing by the trademark owner.
All trademarks and brands within this book are for clarifying purposes only and are the owned by the owners themselves, not affiliated with this document.

TABLE OF CONTENTS

Introduction 1

CHAPTER 1: AYURVEDA AND HISTORY 3

What is Ayurveda? 3
History of Ayurveda 3
The spread of Ayurveda in history 4
Tenets of Ayurveda 4
What makes Ayurveda Unique? 5
Ayurveda respects the "uniqueness" of each individual. 5
Ayurveda considers all the levels of the individual. 5
Ayurveda offers natural ways of treating diseases and promoting health. 6
Ayurveda emphasizes prevention 6
Ayurveda empowers everyone to take responsibility for their well-being 7
Ayurveda is cost-effective. 7
Ayurveda Works 8
Ayurveda - The Ancient Knowledge Of Life 9
Ayurveda - The Allure of Ayurvedic Medicine in the Western World 13
Is Ayurveda a Medical Practice? 13

Isn't Ayurveda based on Science? 13
Ayurvedic Medicine in the Western World 14
Ancient & Modern Ayurveda..............................16
Diet According to Ayurveda 17
Vata Pacifying foods...18
Pitta Pacifying Foods..19
Kapha Pacifying Foods...19

CHAPTER 2: THE SCIENCE OF AYURVEDA 22
Ayurveda - The Science of Life 22
Is Ayurveda Medical Science? 26
Ayurveda - The Science of Medicines and Medical Healing 27
Ayurveda - Age-Old Truth 29
CONCEPT 30
UNIQUENESS...31
PRESENT STATUS 32
PREPARATION...33

CHAPTER 3: AYURVEDA DEVELOPMENT 34
Development of Ayurveda....................................34
Ayurveda & Health - Caring for Body, Mind & Soul..36
Staying Healthy and Happy With Ayurveda 40
Ayurveda Medical Tourism 42

Importance of Ayurveda 43
Ayurveda Help in Tackling Modern Day Problems 46

CHAPTER 4: AYURVEDA AND LIFE.49

How Ayurveda Helps Your Life 49
What Makes Ayurveda So Unique? 51
How Does Ayurveda Work? 51
What Therapies Does Ayurveda Offer? 53
What Does Holistic Mean? 54
Age Gracefully Through Ayurveda 55

CHAPTER 5: AYURVEDA POWER 58

The Unique Power of Ayurveda to Heal Any Health Problem 58
Ayurveda works if someone trusts 58
Why should you switch over to Ayurveda? ...59
7 Beneficial Ayurveda Spices 60
- Black Pepper 61
- Cumin 61
- Cardamom 62
- Coriander 62
- Fennel 63
- Fenugreek 63
- Turmeric 64

CHAPTER 6: AYURVEDA UNTYPICAL TYPES AND SEX 65

Ayurveda - Untypical Types 65

Untypical Types 66

Woman and Childcare in Ayurveda...................67

Ayurveda and Sex...................69

Vageekarana Chikitsa (Aphrodisiac Treatment) 70

Ayurveda and Premature Ejaculation...................71

CHAPTER 7: YOGA AND AYURVEDA .. 73

Yoga Ayurveda - An Introduction to Understanding the Body-Mind-Spirit Connection With Yoga Ayurveda 73

Body Mind Spirit and Yoga Therapy 74

Yoga and Ayurvedic Treatments - A Correlation Between Mind and Body 75

Enhance Your Overall Personality With Ayurveda & Yoga 77

Basic Principles 78

Ayurveda As a Way of Life 79

Ayurveda and Yoga 81

Yoga - The perfect way to perfect health...................82

Eight principles 83

Rules and Regulations 83

Yoga And Prime Ayurvedic Treatments...................87

Ayurveda treatments 88

Yoga Exercises and Ayurveda - Adjusting Your Pace of Yoga Exercises and Yoga Breathing For

Balance 91
Strong Body 91
Stability of Mind 92
Temperature of Body 92
Ayurvedic Yoga Retreats - A Nice Experience With Nature 93
•Selection of the center: 94
•Choosing program: 94
•Accommodation and stay: 95

CHAPTER 8: AYURVEDA AND STRESS 96

Ayurveda - Learn to Cope With Stress 96
Zrii Amalaki And Ayurveda 97
Amalaki Fruit Has Many Health Benefits 98
Beating Stress With Ayurvedic Retreat 99
The Basis for Ayurvedic Treatment for Stress .. 101
•Establish a Balance in your life 102
•Take Adequate Rest 102
•Watch What You Eat 103
•Get Adequate Sleep 103
Can Ayurveda Reduce Medical Costs for Cardiovascular Disease, Stress and Chronic Disorders? 104
5 Ayurvedic Treatments for Natural Stress Reduction 107

Lead a Healthy Lifestyle 107

Opt for a Full Body Massage 108

Meditate 108

Herbal Remedies for Stress....................109

Healthy and Stress-Free Heart by Ayurveda.....110

CHAPTER 9: AYURVEDA HERBS.....114

Tips for Using Ayurveda Herbs to Control Diabetes 114

What is Diabetes? 114

Different Types 115

Common Causes 115

Symptoms 115

Ayurveda and Diabetes 115

Ayurvedic Remedies........................116

Few Ayurvedic Tips for Diabetes 117

Dietary Treatment 118

9 Herbs Benefits in Ayurveda........................119

Common Herbs used in Ayurvedic Medicines.120

*Amalaki (Amla or Indian Gooseberry or Emblica Officinalis) 120

*Ashwagandha (Winter Cherry or Withania Somnifera) 120

*Arjuna (Terminalia Arjuna)........................121

*Guggulu (Shuddha Guggulu, Guggul, Commiphora Mukul) 122

- Karela (Bitter Melon, Bitter Gourd, Momordica Charantia) 122
- Shilajit (Mineral Pitch, Asphaltum) 123
- Triphala (Amalaki, Bibhitaki, Haritaki) 124
- Tulsi (Holy Basil, Ocimum Sanctum) 124

Learning, Teaching and Practicing Ayurveda .. 125

Meditation and Ayurvedic Healing 127

Ayurveda - 7 Distinctive Differences Between Modern and Ayurvedic Medicines 129

- Approach 129
- Side Effects 130
- Natural Treatment 130
- Evidence-Based 130
- Roots 131
- Diet and Lifestyle 132
- Detoxification 132

Your Health And Ayurveda - See The Big Picture, Don't Get Stuck In Details 134

CHAPTER 10: AYURVEDA SOLUTION FOR BETTER SLEEP 137

Ayurvedic Solutions For Better Sleep 137

Ayurvedic Methods for Better Sleep 137

Sukhanidra - Better Sleep With Ayurveda 139

Sleep Therapy - 10 Benefits of Ayurveda 140

- Lemon juice 140

- Having all your senses with you during meals time 141
- Having frequent lunches 141
- Light meals before going to bed 141
- Rest after eating 142
- Keeping yourself well hydrated 142
- Drink lukewarm water laced with aromatic herbs 142
- Meals unaccompanied by ice-drinks 143
- Leaving the day's work at the office 143
- Deep meditation before sleeping 143

How to Cure Insomnia Through Ayurveda? 144

Find Beneficial & Natural Remedies For Insomnia Through Ayurveda 145

Ancient Ayurveda Science and Insomnia 148

Ayurvedic Principles 149

Applying Ayurvedic Principles 150

Ayurveda: A Perfect Cure For Night Discharge Treatment 152

Conclusion 155

INTRODUCTION

Ayurveda is one of the oldest systems of traditional medicine still being practiced. It is a system of holistic health and aims at a combination of diet, medicine and lifestyle changes to bring the body and soul in harmony.

Ayurveda books are regarded as the best means to know the concept of Ayurveda. Ayurveda makes use of various vegetables, minerals, vitamins which are known for its medicinal values. It is regarded as one of the best ways to cure various health problems naturally. Ayurveda books contain the content and methods of preparing various medicines to deal with certain and particular diseases. These books also embrace the character, nature and healing properties of various herbs and natural elements being used in the preparation of ayurvedic medicaments.

Ayurveda books talk about various aspects of Ayurveda such as Ayurveda massage. Ayurvedic massage is a well-known treatment for body disorder and various age-related problems. There are several advantages to taking an ayurvedic massage. Some of them are as follows:

- Gives relief in pain
- Makes muscles flexible
- Improves blood circulation
- Better sleep
- arthritis
- Built a positive attitude towards life
- And various other health benefits.

Ayurveda is a concept which was originated in

India. But, in the present scenario, it is being practiced all over the world as it is a natural way to live a long and healthy life.

Ayurveda books enlighten Ayurveda literature. Ayurveda literature is written by many authors in different languages but the most popular languages are Sanskrit, Hindi, and English. Some of the well known ayurvedic literature is written are Shaligram Nighantu (Sanskrit), banaushadhi chandrodaya (Hindi) and Indian material medica (English).

CHAPTER 1: AYURVEDA AND HISTORY

WHAT IS AYURVEDA?

Ayurveda is derived from two Sanskrit words: "Veda" meaning knowledge and "Ayush" meaning long life. According to the basic tenets of Ayurveda, human life can be prolonged and health improved by following a holistic lifestyle. According to Ayurveda, the prevention of disease is more important than its cure.

HISTORY OF AYURVEDA

The science of Ayurveda is one of the oldest healing sciences that originating in India around 5000 thousand years ago. The belief widely held in India is that the science of healing came about as a divine revelation to Acharya Veda Vyas, who, who put the basic philosophy of Ayurveda in a set of religious books called the Vedas. Significantly, the knowledge contained in the Vedas was taken as true, there have been no instances of testing or experimentation in the treatise.

There were many significant contributors to this body of knowledge over the next 2000 years. Among them was Acharya Charaka, who, in his experience, the Charaka Samhita dated 3 B.C elucidated on immunity, metabolism, and digestion. Acharya Sushruta has recorded instances of surgery on the skull in his treaties, Sushruta Samhita.

With the growth of Hinduism, sages and seers transcribed oral traditions into book form. Ayurveda grew to encompass the use of herbs, colors, foods, aromas, gems, slokas and mantras and even surgery. The Atharva Veda delineated Ayurveda into eight branches and gradually, Ayurveda grew into two schools of medicine:
• Atreya School for Physicians
• Dhanvantari School for Surgeons

The spread of Ayurveda in history
Over the next 1000 years, learners from all over the world came to India to learn about Ayurveda and the spiritual scripts it was recorded in. Travelers from Tibet, China, Greece, Rome, and Persia learned about Ayurveda and took their knowledge of healing back to their countries. Chinese and Unani traditional schools of medicine have their roots in Ayurveda.

Tenets of Ayurveda
Ayurveda is a science that takes into account a person's lifestyle, metabolism, and environment to come up with preventive and curative measures. Each person is a combination of the three principal energies known as Doshas: Kapha, Vata, and Pitta.

One of these energies will be predominant in

each person and accordingly, the diet, medicine, and activity plan would be formulated by the Ayurvedic practitioner to bring the patient's mind and body in harmony.

The physiological makeup and food habits of each person would tend to be Tamsik, Rajsik or Sattvik. Ayurveda is a spiritual science and practices like cleansing, chanting and meditation are prescribed as part of a holistic lifestyle.

WHAT MAKES AYURVEDA UNIQUE?

Ayurveda respects the "uniqueness" of each individual.

The first thing that an Ayurvedic Practitioner will do is determine your mind and body constitution or Prakriti because that will determine the path the treatment will take. Ayurveda believes that no two people are the same even if they have the same constitution. Both patients might have the same ailment but the treatment would be delivered differently or maybe a completely different treatment would be called for.

Ayurveda considers all the levels of the individual.

That means that in Ayurveda we consider the Mind, the Body and the Spirit of an individual. Many times a disease can be in the mind as well as the body and Ayurveda recognize this as they determine the constitution of an individual. Many times an illness will culminate in the mind and the mind is such a powerful thing that the illness will eventually manifest in the body and that is called disease. The disease is the absence of "ease". Ease is a healthy place to be, everyone wants to be at ease.

Ayurveda offers natural ways of treating diseases and promoting health.

Because Ayurveda considers the Mind, the Body and the Spirit of an individual, it focuses on a natural way of being. All things on this planet have varying degrees of the 5 elements which are space, air, fire, water, and earth. Even our bodies are made up of these 5 elements and that is why nature resonates so well with our bodies. That is also the reason that synthetic drugs lose their effectiveness after time, it is because they do not have those 5 elements and without that, they cannot be truly effective in creating health, in many cases they just help with the symptoms and even at times will mask them, however, that is not a cure.

Ayurveda emphasizes prevention.

Ayurveda believes that we have the tools to prevent disease and many of them are inside of us. Our bodies are marvelous machines that act as a pharmacy, we can stay in a state of health just by being conscious of what we eat, our environment, what we see, hear, taste and touch. All of those things contribute to our health but they can also diminish our health as well. It is natural for humans to be in a state of health, the disease is not natural and it is no comfort and it is very preventable.

Ayurveda empowers everyone to take responsibility for their well-being.

Who is our health the most important? Our health is most important to ourselves first and then our loved ones and the people who depend on us. Many times we feel that our doctor is looking at our health as a business and it is a business, it's the business of being a Doctor. I don't mean it is their business, it is a money-making business. Who do you want to be responsible for your well-being, yours or a business? Doctors have their place and that is when you get sick, so what they practice is "sickness" and how to deal with it. When you put your health in your own hands you have a vested interest and you have no gain by being sick. The best policy is to take the best possible care that you can of your self and avoid illness. This responsibility belongs to us, nobody is going to watch out for your health quite the way that you will.

Ayurveda is cost-effective.

The miracle of nature does not have a price tag on it. How much is a life worth? In modern medicine, they say it is worth $50,000 a year and I wonder how they arrived at that number when many medical treatments cost more than that in a month. I think that life is PRICELESS and so does Ayurveda. If we treat our self right by proper nutrition, exercise, positive thinking and paying attention to what we see, touch, taste, hear, smell and feel then we will be in perfect health. There are no injections in Ayurveda so medications are all-natural, directly from nature and delivered in natural ways. Food and herbs are natural, cost-effective and have a great impact on your health.

Ayurveda Works.
Ayurveda has treatments for things that modern medicine has classified as "untreatable" or "un-curable". Ayurveda takes a standpoint that nothing is un-treatable or un-curable it may be that we don't know how to treat it or how to cure it just yet but there will be a treatment or a cure so it is our job to support the body and the mind until that can be found. Ayurveda can cure hepatitis C and that is not something that is easily done in Western medicine, not even by transplanting the liver. Ayurveda is now being recognized by modern medicine because of some of the impressive results that have been realized by Ayurvedic treatments.

Ayurveda emphasized the importance of maintaining positive health. Not only maintaining it but creating it as well, Ayurveda focuses on preventing the imbalances that lead to disease. An individualized and multi-dimensional approach is taken for the prevention of disease as well as for treatment.

AYURVEDA - THE ANCIENT KNOWLEDGE OF LIFE

Widely regarded as the oldest form of health care in the world, Ayurveda is an intricate holistic medical system, lifestyle, and philosophy that originated in India and Sri Lanka some 5,000 to 7,000 years ago.

Ayurveda is a Sanskrit word, consisting of two different words - Ayu and Veda, the literal translation of which is Knowledge of Life. Ayurveda is a part of the Atharva Veda, one of the four Vedas in Hindu Philosophy, and is also known as Asthanga Veda.

Some people may be concerned that you need to become religious to adopt the principles of Ayurveda, but this is not the case.

The principles of Ayurveda are an invaluable link to understanding, in detail, naturally healthy living.

Every medical science has some basic principles on which the structure of the science is built and fabricated. The principles of Ayurveda are based on nature and the Vedic philosophy of healthy living and are very simple to understand.

Following the principles of Ayurveda brings about a profound understanding of the inner ability to have sound body, mind, and spirit. The basic principles of Ayurveda state that the world of matter arises from an underlying non-material field known as consciousness.

Ayurveda sees everything in the universe, including human beings, as being composed of five basic elements: space, air, fire, water, and earth. Any part of the body, however minuscule, is an inseparable combination of these principles.

The principles of Ayurveda are based on the concept of Tridosha, or the system of three Doshas: Vata, Pitta, and Kapha. A proper understanding of Tridosha is the basis of Ayurveda's knowledge.

Dosha types are the classifications used in the practice and study of Ayurveda to categorize the primary body-mind personalities. Dosha means "that which changes".

While every individual has aspects of each Dosha in their constitution, Ayurveda determines the influence of each of these on a numeric scale. Every person has a different mixture of Doshas; usually, one Dosha is predominant, and another is secondary.

Generally, Vata is the controlling Dosha, Pitta is the changing Dosha, and Kapha is the making Dosha.

Discovering your Dosha is the first and most important step you can take on a personal health care program. We must determine our Dosha, or combination of Doshas, to determine which foods, drinks, and lifestyle patterns best fit our constitution.

The best way to accurately determine your Dosha

is to consult an Ayurvedic doctor, but there are other, easier ways to get a good idea of what Dosha you are.

Firstly, you could use one of many free online Dosha tests. Secondly, you could use PC software such as the Ayurveda Almanac, which provides a much more thorough assessment, with recommendations for diet, as well as providing you with a means to identify early signs of many diseases.

Ayurvedic medicine provides a clear, concise, cohesive regimen to enhance the health of your mind and body in a natural, holistic way. Ayurvedic texts emphasize ahara (proper diet) as vital for promoting health and happiness.

Diagnosis according to Ayurveda is to find out the root cause of a disease, and diseases reflect the predominant Dosha that produces them.

Negative health may arise from an imbalance in the three Doshas - and the science of Ayurveda is used to bring back this essential harmony. Each herb, food, drink, and even environment contains Dosha characteristics so using the opposite to balance out an individual is done in Ayurveda.

But for subtler imbalances, the principles of Ayurveda can help you respond in simple ways to restore balance sooner rather than later.

Ayurveda is a journey to perfect health, peace of mind and, ultimately, to enlightenment, and is merely about making healthy choices in daily life. It is a science that teaches you how to live in a true and natural balance.

Ayurveda is one of many Alternative Medicines

that are being used today. Ayurveda is considered a complete, holistic way of life, rather than just medical science. Ayurveda is the healing side of Yoga, and Yoga is the spiritual side of Ayurveda. It must be emphasized that Ayurveda is not a substitute for Western allopathic medicine. Ayurveda is not only a system of medicine but also a way of healthy living.

AYURVEDA - THE ALLURE OF AYURVEDIC MEDICINE IN THE WESTERN WORLD

Ayurveda is an ancient medical practice native to India whose prevalence in the Western world finds a foothold in the last three decades. While there is an obvious attraction to Ayurvedic medicine in the western world, one can always find skeptics who wouldn't even consider educating themselves on the subject before rushing to judgment.

Is Ayurveda a Medical Practice?
No. Ayurveda is not a medical practice, which is in contrast to the prevalent notion in the West. Ayurveda is akin to 'herbalism'. Herbalism is the ancient practice of finding natural cures for human maladies which goes back 60,000 years when the Neanderthal men depended on nature's herbs to cure human sicknesses as well as attend to their animals' health issues.
As civilizations started developing in China, Greece, and India, the inhabitants started following different forms of herbalism, which is now known in India as 'Ayurveda'.

Isn't Ayurveda based on Science?
It is a common misconception in the western world that since Ayurveda is thought of as

alternative medicine, it is non-scientific. Often Ayurveda is thought of as an exotic practice enjoyed in health spas. The Sanskrit word Ayurveda is made of two words: Ayur, meaning life and Veda, meaning knowledge. In other words, Ayurveda is a logical and systematic arrangement of herbal knowledge; it's the science of life that encompasses mind, body, and spirit.

AYURVEDIC MEDICINE IN THE WESTERN WORLD

As mentioned before, Ayurvedic medicine has become popular in the western world in the last two or three decades. Many universities now offer courses in alternative medicine practice and many people have begun to treat it as a mainstream career option.
The allure of Ayurveda is mainly because of its nature of the treatment. There are two main aims of Ayurvedic medicine:
"It treats the symptoms of a disease and it helps individuals to strengthen their immune system. Ayurveda treats the body, mind, and spirit of a person as a whole entity, and works on the basis that the mind and body affect each other, and together can overcome disease".
In other words, Ayurvedic medicine believes in holistic healing. Unlike conventional or western medicine which begins treatment only when a

human body contacts an ailment, Ayurveda begins healing before any diseases take place. This is preventive medicine in its purest form.

Ayurvedic herbs can be found in almost every household in India. Hence, the children are surrounded by the preventive nature of the herbs right from the beginning, which lessens the intensity with which diseases are contracted. Let's take a small example - in any western country chances are that someone suffering from the common cold will rush to the doctor or the nearest medical center for treatment. In Asian countries, you will seldom find people visiting the clinic just to treat the same condition. The Ayurvedic remedies for the same condition are a pinch of turmeric mixed with a glass of milk, a teaspoon of honey and a few drops of lime juice.

It is true that people in Asian countries also suffer from major health problems but their focus is always on holistic cure rather than short-term solutions that western medicines provide. The preventive nature of Ayurveda, or rather its curative nature, is the prime reason why western researchers are increasingly allured by Ayurveda.

ANCIENT & MODERN AYURVEDA

Ayurveda is a transnational phenomenon in the 21st century whose wide range of perspective incorporates the economic, socio-political, anthropological, philosophical, pharmacological and biomedical responses.

In the recent past, a dichotomy between the classical (ancient) and modern Ayurveda was created. Ayurvedic experts, practitioners, and researchers classify the 'ancient' Ayurvedic wisdom as the original. 'Modern' Ayurveda to them is that very same knowledge which has been exported from the East to the West, where it was modified. reinterpreted and then was re-imported to Eastern countries.

Yet, there are still many who feel that this is simply an ideological difference. Some would argue that the western world which is so attuned to giving importance to things based on its "provable" value backed by scientific research is trying to modernize Ayurveda too on the same grounds.

To any practitioner of Ayurveda, this is an unjustified and unimportant addition to Ayurvedic medicine because a healing system that is based on the natural healing processes endowed by Mother Nature itself cannot be confined into scientific proportions.

Nevertheless, the allure of Ayurveda remains a predominant factor in the acceptance of the same in the western world because of its natural and preventive healing measures.

DIET ACCORDING TO AYURVEDA

Ayurveda also insists that the dietary needs of every individual are different and hence specific body constitutions need a specific diet. The importance is given to diet and nutrition in the Ayurveda system of medicine, then, cannot be underestimated. The conversion of food in nutrition is called Agni or fire in Ayurveda. A vegetarian diet is always preferred over a non-vegetarian diet. Ayurveda suggests that an individual's diet should contain rich amounts of vegetables, fruits, whole grains and foods rich in fiber as these will provide energy and help the individual maintain good health.

A good meal as suggested by Ayurveda would also include colors, aromas, flavors, tastes, textures, etc that would soothe all our sense organs apart from providing our body with all the needed nutrients. Ayurveda discourages the use of animal flesh in our diet as also the consumption of coffee and alcohol.

Herbs and spices do play a vital part in all Ayurveda diets and recipes. Ayurveda suggests that one consume herbs before a meal, during a meal and after a meal. vitamins etc. Herbs are known to increase the digestion process and help in the assimilation of food due to their ability to transport the healing and nutritive value of food to the tissues, cells, and organs. Herbs also cleanse our body system of toxins and impurities and help in the process of elimination.

Eating a lemon before a meal increases the

appetite as also chewing fennel seeds after a meal helps in the digestive process and makes our breath fresher. Amalakhi rasayanas and Triphala Rasayana are highly recommended in Ayurveda as these help digestion, assimilation, and elimination. The best way to consume spices is by consuming them after cooking. Ayurveda favors the inclusion of all the six tastes: sweet, sour, salty, astringent, bitter and pungent at every meal. These easy to digest recipes offer quick assimilation, prevent diseases, provide immunity from diseases, impart improved sleep and concentration, maintain youthfulness and offer energy, strength, and vitality to an individual. The Ayurveda system of medicine recommends suitable and unsuitable types of food for each category of body constitution. These are to be followed for a long and healthy life free from diseases. The food consumed by a person should have relevance to his body constitution. Ayurveda recommends foods based on the doshas of each person and what type of food is beneficial for each body type.

Vata Pacifying foods.
Vata pacifying foods include ghee, soft dairy products, wheat, rice, corn, and bananas. It is recommended that a person with a Vata constitution consume foods like hot cereal with ghee, soups, vegetables, cooked grains, chapattis, etc. Unlike other body constitution persons, Vata persons can consume spicy foods as well.

Vegetables: Asparagus, carrots, cucumber, green beans, onions, garlic, turnips, radish, sweet potatoes, etc Fruits Mangoes, melons, peaches, bananas and all sweet fruits Grains Rice, wheat and oats.

Pitta Pacifying Foods.
For people with a pitta constitution, milk, rice, beans, and fruits as also spices such as cumin, coriander is recommended. Vegetables: There are no restrictions on the consumption of vegetables by the pita constitution persons. They can generally consume all types of vegetables. Fruits: There are also no restrictions on the type of fruits that they consume. All fruits are generally good for them.

Kapha Pacifying Foods.
And for Kapha dosha persons, foods with bitter, pungent and astringent tastes are beneficial. Foods such as puffed rice, millets, and leafy vegetables as also spices such as ginger, turmeric, and chili are good for Kapha constitution persons.
Vegetables: All vegetables are god for these persons. But if some of these Kapha persons suffer from diseases such as asthma, lung congestion, heart disease, obesity, etc then, it would be best to avoid sweet juicy vegetables like cucumbers, sweet potatoes, etc Grains: Rice, wheat, millets, etc are recommended. In the Ayurveda system of medicine, apart from consuming the type of food suitable for each

dosha type, the seasons and the place where one life is also taken into consideration. Ayurveda diet, stresses the importance of consuming whole foods, eaten in as natural a state as possible. And it is also to be noted that if the digestive fire is not strong enough, then, even wholesome foods can turn into the toxic matter in the body.

Ayurveda system of medicine does not recommend foods that are frozen, canned or refined as these dilute the food of its nutritive value. Also to be avoided are processed foods with artificial colors, flavorings, additives or preservatives. Also, foods that are genetically altered and grown with the use of chemical fertilizers and pesticides are not favored in Ayurveda. The best option, then, would be to consume foods that are organic, natural and locally available. Ayurveda also stresses the importance of rotation of an individual's diet so that one does not consume the same type of food every day of the week. There should always be variety in the types of food consumed as this will provide us with all the needed nutrients, increase the digestion process as also it will increase one's liking for every type of food.

Food Intake -Do's and Don'ts. Certain guidelines have been suggested in Ayurveda regarding the dietary habits that should help an individual maintain good health, nourish the body and balance the **doshas.**

- One should always consume cooked foods and avoid raw foods.
- Fruits and salad vegetables, however, can be

eaten raw.
- The food consumed should neither be too hot or too cold.
- Curds are recommended after a heavy meal as it helps digestion.
- One should always chew one's food properly.
- One should wash the hands, feet, and face before every meal.
- Food should be consumed only if the bowel movements are proper.
- There should always be a gap of three hours between every meal.
- It is advisable to have a heavy lunch; however, a light dinner is recommended.
- One should always limit the intake of food to two-thirds of the stomach capacity.

The following food combinations are best avoided:
- Never consume milk and meat
- Starchy foods such as potatoes and fruits should not be taken together.

Note:

It is to be noted that this information is purely for educational purposes and is not intended to diagnose, treat, cure or prevent any disease. Please consult your Ayurveda physician for all your specific dietary needs.

CHAPTER 2: THE SCIENCE OF AYURVEDA

AYURVEDA - THE SCIENCE OF LIFE

Lord Brahma, the creator according to Hindu mythology created this earth in six days. It included plants, animals and natural resources. But as time progressed there were lots of miseries on earth and people were sufferings with so many diseases. Seeing this Brahma- the Creator laid the foundation of Ayurveda, which slowly descended to earth.

Ayurveda means the science of life. This is a science that not only deals with the treatment of the diseased condition but also teaches us the various methodologies that are essential to carry out a healthy and happy living. These methods are time tested and uncountable people have gained extreme benefits from wonders of Ayurveda.

As Ayurveda has a divine origin, it is considered a holistic science that is blessed by God. Some of the various sages have contributed their whole life in spreading the magic of Ayurveda in this world that is suffering from various ailments and sorrows. The main motto behind spreading this divine knowledge was to make people achieve the contented life essential for healthy and peaceful livings.

Besides roaming as nomads to spread the knowledge, they wrote many books. Books like

Charka Samhita, Susruta Samhita, and Ashtanga samgraha are considered as the pillars of the ayurvedic world. These books or the encyclopedias of Ayurveda contain invaluable knowledge that is made after extensive researches made by these genius sages.

Many people doubt that Ayurveda might just be an observatory science and bear no scientific backdrop. But it is a big myth. Ayurveda thought an observatory science, also bears a deep scientific explanation of all the procedures and suggestions that are mentioned by it. Medical sciences are getting surprised with the results they are getting today after extensive researches to prove the worth of Ayurveda. It is quite astonishing that those sages carried out such a deep study about our body and functioning of various organs of our body without having any facilities and sophisticated instruments to aid there searches. They applied the fundamentals of Vata, pitta and Kapha and the five Mahabharata concepts to carry out their research.

Ayurveda consist of eight parts, these are known as Asht-aang (eight parts). These are as follows.
- Medicine (kaya chikitsa)
- Surgery (shalya chikitsa)
- ENT and eye (Chanakya chikitsa)
- Psychiatry (bhoot vidya)
- Pediatrics (Baal tantra)
- Toxicology (agad tantra)
- Science of rejuvenation (Rasayana)
- Aphrodisiac life (bajikarana or vajikarana)

Charka Samhita, the manual of medicine has

been originally written by Acharya Agnivesha. After getting oral teaching from his preacher Punarvasu Atrey in the form of verses, he composed a book named as Agnivesha Tantra. This Agnivesha Tantra was then revised by Maharishi Charka and this eventually became famous. This book is presently known as Charka Samhita.

This book contains 8 chapters named as
- **Su**tra sthana
- Nidan sthana
- Vimana sthana
- Sharira sthana
- Indriya sthana
- Chikitsa sthana
- Kalpa sthana
- Siddhi sthana

Charka Samhita is not just a medicinal or a treatment book; it also explains the ways to increase the living standards and to attain a lifestyle that will keep you away from sorrows and miseries. According to Charka Samhita, Ayurveda has two basic principles
- To maintain the health of a healthy individual
- To treat a diseased person.

The complete ayurvedic world works on these two lines, to give support to the people devastated from there miseries (both physical and mental).

Besides these, Charka Samhita also contains a detailed explanation of various herbs used in preparing ayurvedic medicines. As Ayurveda is based on the remedies provided by natural

resources (plant and animal sources), Charka mentioned everything about them in detail. Even the methods of taking them as medicine or as food are also mentioned separately in a well explanatory fashion. Various regimens are also present that tend to make you disease-free and socially acclaimed. These are divided into four categories. These are
- Day regimen
- Night regimen
- Diet regimen
- Behavioral regimen.

The focus of Ayurveda is not just on the growth of an individual but also to work for the upliftment of the whole society to make it a better place to live.

Ayurveda also contains detailed methods of examining a patient, various examinations like tenfold examination, 8 fold examination, and 3 fold examinations are done to reach a consensus and to diagnose the cause of a disease. The wonder of panchakarma is also a gift of Ayurveda that is very famous in the western part of this world.

So long but yet so short. Ayurveda is endless. Even to define Ayurveda in an article is a very difficult job. This article carries a brief idea that Ayurveda wants to present to this world. The world of Ayurveda is full of happiness and peace. Let us come together to explore this beautiful gift that Mother Nature has left for us. Come and join hands with Ayurveda and the real pleasure of healthy living.

IS AYURVEDA MEDICAL SCIENCE?

Ayurveda might be defined as an important complementary medical practice developed by Hindu and Brahma cultures and which was initiated about 2 millenniums ago. It is worth pouting out that Ayurveda changed and incorporated values form different cultures. Since it has been named the science of life, Ayurveda tries to restore the connections between natural resources and human beings. This science depends on the values of nature and of the universe. Herbal medicine might be considered an important practice within Ayurveda. All the elements of the universe are vital resources for the human body and the spirit. Ayurveda might be defined as the science of the five elements (air, earth, ether, water, and fire) simply because this practice considers that a healthy life depends on the inner and outer equilibrium that these elements provide.

Ayurveda pays attention to emotional manifestations therefore, any kind of disharmony might be solved with the help of Ayurveda beliefs. Healthy diets stand for valuable methods to preserve the equilibrium that we already talked about. Ayurveda practices are established depending on a special diagnosis, which interprets holistically physical and mental manifestations, in terms of five elements of the cosmos.

Ayurveda's values and beliefs rely on a constant healthy lifestyle.

Ayurveda is a sort of complementary practice, which outlines the importance of connections we create with the universe. The human body is not isolated from the universal values, on the contrary, it is part of the universe, and might be considered its sixth element.

AYURVEDA - THE SCIENCE OF MEDICINES AND MEDICAL HEALING

The process of Ayurveda is the oldest healing process in the world. Ayurveda massage symbolizes the cycle of Life or Science with the study of Longevity. Ayurveda provides you the medical treatments for physical and psychological ailments. These massages include herbs and herbal medicines, medical massages, oil treatments, and body cleansing therapy. The treatment processes are all-natural and have no side effects. The Ayurveda go deeply to the root cause of the illness rather than the symptoms and provides lasting effects rather than temporary relief.

The Ayur Yog features principles of
- Ayurveda
- Panchakarma
- Kerala ayurvedic massage,

The ayurvedic facilities in Kerala are in medicated oils and herbs.

In south India, karela has been the most

traditional way and its base of the Ayurvedic oil massage therapies. It has modified many techniques to suit the needs of a person who is diseased and to cure them completely.

These therapy processes are known today as the Kerala special treatments and include various elements like:-
- Abhyangam
- Shirodhara
- Shirovasti
- Pichu
- Pizhichil
- Navarakkizhi
- Talam etc.

There are indoor treatments facilities which are provided in Kerala including the
- + Ayurvedic clinics
- + Hospitals
- + Nursing home
- + Resorts
- + Retreats

That can take care of the needs and expectations of all. The Ayurveda in India translates into a more efficient way that is the Science of Life here Ayur symbolizes life and Veda symbolizes the science. Ayurveda is the oldest and very much developed life science of the healing in the world naturally. Life is an important part of the human body that is made up of and for various links that are:-
- Body(shareer),
- sense organs (Indriya),
- Psyche (Mana)

- Soul (Atma).

Ayurveda is not exactly a system of Healing, but a smoothing way of life that only aims to bring about the perfect balance of the entire personality including the body, mind, and spirit all together. Ayurveda is a therapy that is based on the theory of tridosha of the three Biological forces that is the Vata, Pitta, and Kapha. The disease normally arises when there is a mental and physical imbalance among the three Doshas in the body and the therapy aims to bring about the required equilibrium to make the person well balanced.

AYURVEDA - AGE-OLD TRUTH

Ayurvedic medicine, an ancient Indian healing system is right in sync with our growing awareness of the mind-body connection and places equal emphasis on body, mind, and spirit and strives to restore the innate harmony of the individual.

CONCEPT

The basic concept of Ayurvedic medicine is that the body is seen as a microcosmic universe in which the five primordial elements (panchamahabhutas) - ether (akasha), air (Vayu), fire (Agni), water (Jala) and earth (Prithvi) - combine to form three senses of humor (doshas), known as wind (Vata), choler (pitta) and phlegm (Kapha). It's believed each dosha has its qualities and functions about the body.

The balance between these doshas determines the individual constitution (Prakriti) and predisposition to the disease. The constitution is also affected by the strength of a person's 'digestive fire' (Agni) and bowel function (kostha). Seven tissues (dhatus) and their waste products (malas) make up the physical body and a network of channels circulate fluids and essences around the body. Three interdependent universal constituents, the three Gunas - purity (sattva), activity (rajas) and solidity (tamas) - also influence health and determine mental qualities.

The disease occurs if lifestyle, mental or external factors cause an imbalance in one or more of these components. Ayurvedic medicine treats the majority of its patients using herbal mixtures, other organic food, and substances that have been clinically tested and are now being scientifically validated.

UNIQUENESS

Its uniqueness lies in its treatment plan which is tailored to the body type and individual imbalances among the Vata, pitta, and Kapha within and includes dietary changes, exercise, yoga, meditation, massage, herbal tonics, herbal sweat baths, medicated enemas, and medicated inhalations.

Ayurvedic medicine gets rid of the body of its indigestible toxins which attract viruses and compromise autoimmune processes and responses. Ayurvedic physicians pay close attention to pulse, tongue, eyes, and nails in diagnosing illness. Diagnosis is based on observation rather than laboratory testing. The doctor enquires the patient about his health and family histories. Also, he may palpate the body, or listen to the heart, lungs, and intestines with a stethoscope. He uses urine samples and the pulse to describe the balance (or imbalance) of the three doshas. Ayurvedic treatment then consists of cleansing and detoxification (Shodan or Pancha Karma), palliation (Shaman) to balance and relax the three doshas, rejuvenation (Rasayana), and mental hygiene and spiritual healing (Satvajaya)

PRESENT STATUS

At present, Ayurveda medicine is well set to re-orient itself to modern scientific parameters. Simultaneously, it is well poised for much greater, effective utilization to benefit the whole humanity to reach its goals of Health. Ayurveda medicine which started as a magico-religious practice matured into a fully developed medical science with eight branches which have parallels in the modern western system of medicine and it has developed into following sixteen specialties

- Ayurveda Siddhanta (Fundamental Principals of Ayurveda).
- Ayurveda Samhita.
- Rachna Sharira (Anatomy).
- Kriya Sharira (Physiology).
- Dravya Guna Vigian (Materia Medica & Pharmacology).
- Ras-Shastra.
- Bhaishajya Kalpana (Pharmaceuticals).
- Kaumar Bharatiya (Pediatrics).
- Prasuti Tantra (Obstetrics & Gynaecology).
- Swasth-Vritla (Social & Preventive Medicine).
- Kayachikitsa (Internal Medicine).
- Rog Nidan (Pathology).
- Shalya Tantra (Surgery
- Shalkya Tantra (Eye & ENT).
- Mano-Roga (Psychiatry)
- Panchkarma.

PREPARATION

The main part of Ayurveda Medicine is Herbal Tonics or Rasayanas which are prepared according to the Vedic traditional standards practiced in ancient times. They are made of only 100% natural ingredients, using only the best of the Ayurveda and Western herbs and spices, ghee (purified butter), raw honey, dried fruits, Sucanat (unprocessed sugar) and natural flavors. They are prepared by hand (the old custom), using utensils of copper, iron, and clay. Being highly nutritious and antioxidant they provide many elements that are lacking in the modern diet. formulated to bring back into balance one or more of the five elements, which get put out of balance from improper diet etc. In return, this promotes balance on the physical, mental and subtle levels of our being which will add life to our years as well as years to your life.

CHAPTER 3: AYURVEDA DEVELOPMENT

DEVELOPMENT OF AYURVEDA

According to Indian mythology, the origin of Ayurveda has a link with Brahma, the God of Creation. If the mythologies are to be believed, the Hindu myths say that Brahma wanted to erase the suffering of humans by offering knowledge of Ayurveda to other Gods. To do so, he passed on this knowledge to Dhanvantari - father of Ayurveda. He then transmitted the knowledge to the mortal sages so that they could heal their sufferings. It is because of all these myths associated with Ayurveda, that it is considered as a divine science of revelation and thus values personal insight as much as an empirical observation.

As far as the development of Ayurveda is concerned, it is believed that the birth of Indian medicine can be traced back to the days of the famous Indus - Valley civilization of 2700-1500B.C. We note that mythico - religious hymns related to the civilization written in Sanskrit are mentioned in holy books, the Vedas. There are four Vedas, and out of these four Vedas, Arthavaveda; the youngest one provides us with the knowledge of medical practices of Ayurveda. The Golden Age of Ayurveda was from 800 - 1000B.C. This period is marked as the evolution of medical science in India.

Ayurveda flourished significantly during the times of Buddha (520B.C.). Many unique formulas such as mixing mercury, sulfur and different metals with beneficial herbs in medical composition were invented by the Ayurveda practitioners during this period. Nagarjuna, the Buddhist herbologist was the greatest exponent of medical science during that period. Ayurveda practitioners such as Nagbodhi, Yashodhana, Govinda, and Vagbhatta worked along with him during that period. The tradition of Ayurveda went on from centuries to centuries and was passed on from one generation to another.

The Ayurvedic process of treatment has gained popularity in the west too. Even people in the west have started practicing the tradition of Ayurveda to heal and enhance the longevity of the healed. After the independence of India in 1947, Ayurveda was recognized as an official form of medicine along with allopathic, homeopathy, naturopathy, Unani, Tibb, Siddha and yoga therapy. Now we have Ayurvedic Universities in Jamnagar, Gujrat, and Bhubaneswar which conduct research and higher education in Ayurveda. Many doctors are practicing Ayurveda and using the Ayurvedic method of treatment through medicines. The Ayurvedic medicines and its method of treatment are even considered to be safe as they do not have any side-effects on the human body.

AYURVEDA & HEALTH - CARING FOR BODY, MIND & SOUL

The entire cosmos has originated from the basic substances - The Panchmahabhutas (Sky, Air, Fire, Water & Earth). Ayurveda - The world's oldest science of healing, is the Divine-largess to humanity, for health and beauty care, is derived from the four principal Vedas: the Rig Veda, Yajur Veda, Sama Veda, and the Atharva Veda. It is not an alternative but the original science of healing, known to this world, which originated in the Indian subcontinent about 5000 years ago. Ayurveda is derived from two words, ayu (age & life) & Veda (encyclopedia) and 'Charak Samhita' (An ancient Ayurvedic epic), expands upon this definition, telling us that ayu is the "combination of the body, sense organs, mind and soul", the factors responsible for preventing decay.

The Divine creation of the eternal macrocosm is the most precious Divine gift and Life is its quintessence of which Ayurveda provides a complete description. The Vedic science of Ayurveda that deals with the principles and practices of the ways of healthy & happy living, claims Prakriti (nature) and Purusha (The man) as the root factors behind the creation of the world. Man is considered as a boon of nature, the supreme, who in himself bears all the characteristics of his originator and the ability to procreate. As a thesaurus of health, Ayurveda provides basic intellectual elements and principles of medicine, very minutely.

Ayurveda was based perfectly on empirical observations & practice rather than philosophy alone. The traditional medicines used in Ayurveda are of herbal, mineral & animal origin whose efficacy has already been proven, scientifically now. The "Perfect Health Philosophy" of Ayurveda believes and proposes that he who is in the habit of taking balanced & suitable food comprising of all essential nutritional elements, leads a perfect and happy life. The entire system of Ayurvedic treatment is based on correcting & balancing of Tridoshas (The three senses of humor or the blemishes or the metabolic components of the body), Sapta-Dhatus (The seven physical elements of the body or the vital components) and Malas (The end product of elimination or the bodily excreta), which when get excited or vitiated, due to exogenous or endogenous causes including deficiency of nutritional ingredients, result in the impairment of body functions or disease. It may be trite but certainly a true remark that "we start dying the day we are born". The decay and degeneration, causing discomfort, disorder, disease or debility and ultimately culminating in the death of the organism, are a part and parcel of our biological being. Charak Samhita signifies "Only that, which can bring about a cure, is true medicine and only that who can relieve his patients of their ailments is the true physician" (Sutrasthanam, Chapter-I, Verse 134).

Even an acute poison can become an excellent drug if it is properly processed & administered and on the other hand, even the most outstanding drug, if not properly processed & administered, becomes an acute poison.

Health & Ayurveda: At its simplest, HEALTH is the absence of physical and mental diseases. W.H.O. makes the description wider by adding that "All people should have the opportunity to fulfill their genetic potential". This includes the ability to grow and develop physically and mentally without the impediments of inadequate nutrition or environment contamination and to be protected as much as possible against infectious diseases.

Ayurveda had made this concept of Health even wider (centuries ago) by describing Health as the perfect state of well-being of the organism when it functions optimally without evidence of disease or abnormality besides the balancing of Physical, Physiological, Psychological, Sentimental & Spiritual functionings of a living body.

According to Ayurveda, Debility can be described as generalized weakness and lack of energy, vigor or strength, which may be caused by various Physical or Physiological disorders. And when associated with Psychological, Sentimental or Spiritual-disorders, it also represents a lack of desire or ambition and loss of power or sensation along with non-specific symptoms like fatigability, insomnia, drowsiness, lethargy, unwanted anxiety, loss of appetite, lack of interest in personal or family matters, etc.. All the cheerful pleasures of nature's greatest, priceless gift of Human life are solely dependent on the perfect state of health. And in today's scientific & mechanical era of Space-age, the load of work & problems is increasing every moment which is getting burdensome & tiresome day by day, leading ultimately towards a dull life associated with unwanted debilities.

The fundamental concept of Ayurveda, emphasizes that a perfectly balanced diet containing all essential nutrients plays a vital role in maintaining a perfect state of health. The basis of a good diet is variety because none of a single food contains all nutrients essential for Health. Ayurveda has stored in its vast treasure, a wide range of herbal formulations to supplement the nutritional deficiencies for maintaining a perfect state of health and fulfill the desires of Longevity.

Interestingly, without forgetting the principles of nature and theories of natural constitution, Ayurveda suggests in numerous recipes to supplement the body with such essential nutritional ingredients available from nature's resources for the cure of or protection from diseases, because the basic motive of Ayurveda is to treat & cure the ailing & suffering and maintain the health of healthy human beings. Truly speaking, treating with Ayurveda means worshiping nature.

STAYING HEALTHY AND HAPPY WITH AYURVEDA

Ayurveda health spas around the world are offering the secret to health and happiness once reserved for the royal families of ancient India. For thousands of years, Ayurveda, the original health science of India, recommended panchakarma treatments regularly as the key to health and happiness.

Panchakarma means "the five actions" -- a routine of massage, herbal steam baths, and other measures to detoxify the body. Ayurveda holds that eliminating impurities allows the body's channels to be open for the free flow of nature's intelligence - which also means the flow of bliss in the body. Rogers Badgett, the owner of an ayurvedic spa in Fairfield, IA, observes, "There is a flow of intelligence -- a communication -- between every cell and organ in the body and this is what maintains optimal functioning of the mind and body. According to Ayurveda, true health is a state of balance that produces bliss as well as vitality. Health and happiness go hand in hand."

The effect of happiness on health is well accepted. We all know the saying, "laughter is the best medicine." Modern science has shown that emotions stimulate neuropeptides, which are immuno-modulators. These bind to receptors in the kidneys, heart, and liver - in fact, all over the body. At the same time, organs have been found to produce their neuropeptides, which bind back with the brain. The whole body can be seen as a communication network. This supports the Ayurvedic perspective that happiness is a two-way street: happiness creates health and health create happiness. One can see why the world's most ancient system of healthcare, Ayurveda, recommends regular panchakarma treatments. When toxins and impurities disrupt the natural flow of intelligence in the body -- it disrupts the communication system of the body -- health and happiness are affected. Complications arise and the once-perfect mind/body system begins to suffer. Eliminate the blockages and the body once more returns to optimal health.

A full Panchakarma treatment program at an Ayurveda health spa usually begins with a consultation with ayurvedic experts who use the ancient technique of pulse assessment to determine body type, one's level of imbalance and where the imbalances are located. Based on the assessment, an individualized panchakarma program is then created to soften and eliminate impurities and to target specific areas where blockages and toxic buildup has occurred.

Although Ayurveda offers a wide spectrum of specialized rejuvenation treatments. Most Ayurveda spa treatment programs do not isolate any one treatment modality over any other. A full week's rejuvenation treatment plan typically includes at least 6 or 7 different treatments. The various treatments are meant to work together synergistically in a holistic regimen to remove blockages to the natural flow of the body's intelligence. Where the blockage is and what quality (or dosha) is associated with the blockage determines the location and *q*uality of symptom that is being experienced. But, according to Ayurveda, the underlying cause of the symptom is that the flow of intelligence, bliss, or consciousness has been blocked. This is why Ayurveda spas can address a wide range of symptoms and disorders through the individualized purification and detoxification therapies of panchakarma.

AYURVEDA MEDICAL TOURISM

Ayurveda Medical Tourism is traveling to India to avail of various Ayurvedic therapies. Medical Tourism for Ayurveda can be planned either to cure diseases or to rejuvenate and revitalize the body that helps in maintaining optimum health. There are hundreds of thousands of tourists and travelers that come to India for ayurvedic treatments for their various stubborn health ailments not responded to other medicines and therapies.

Unlike mainstream medicinal science, Ayurveda does not use any chemical or synthetic based products and hence, ayurvedic medicines are considered to be one of the safest medications in the world. You can find a lot of information about Ayurveda dosha, Ayurveda Panchakarma treatments and many more topics on the internet that play a significant role in diagnosing and treating the diseases.

Nevertheless, there are plenty of Ayurveda health centers that just attract tourists and provide no effective treatments. Being a foreigner, you must find an authentic Ayurveda treatment center that gets you promising results. You can find a qualified ayurvedic doctor who can advise you about where to find such genuine Ayurveda panchakarma centers. This saves you from ending up in complications of the diseases due to poor or improper treatments prescribed and performed by quacks.

Ayurvedadosha is one of the trusted and tested places where you can find all information about Ayurveda including Medical Tourism in India for Ayurveda. You can personally mail mentioning your health ailment and ask for the help. You can find the best economical Ayurveda panchakarma center in India that can save your money without compromising the quality.

IMPORTANCE OF AYURVEDA

Ayurveda has been widely recognized as a system of natural health care congenial to the health needs of women. All over the world, more and more women are turning to herbal medicine so that they have total control of their bodies throughout the year, throughout their lives. Vedas are the ancient books of knowledge, or science, from India. They contain practical and scientific information on various subjects beneficial to humanity like health, philosophy, engineering, astrology, etc. Ayurveda helps women find their body rhythm, which is closely linked with nature and its changes resulting in lasting solutions to their health problems.

As women respond both mentally and physically better to Ayurveda, it is known as a women's health care system. Ayurveda gives equal importance to mental health for which a regime of ethical life (sadurutta) is prescribed. Ayurveda is the science of life. Ayurveda is a science dealing not only with the treatment of some diseases but is a complete way of life. Strict mental discipline and strict adherence to moral values are considered a pre-requisite for mental health. Finally, herbs that are pungent, bitter and astringent ameliorate Kapha-water, which means they tend to increase digestive fire, expel and dry excessive fluid build up in the system, including clearing excessive fat from the body, and the accumulation of cholesterol and other fatty deposits in the veins and arteries of the body.

Ayurveda had recognized the importance of the environment in total health. Remember, everything in your environment is composed of doshas that interact with your doshas. Ayurvedic health care enhances the results of Yoga. Ayurvedic healthcare is the best bet for women to stop the aging process. Periodic rejuvenation therapy will keep health, beauty, and zest for life intact throughout the years. Ayurveda gives equal importance to mental health for which a regime of ethical life is prescribed. Herbs that have pungent, sour and salty flavors stimulate fire; herbs that are astringent (drying) and bitter stimulate Vata-air or the nerve centered humor; herbs that are sweet, salty and sour stimulate or increase Kapha-water or the mucoid humor. Strict mental discipline and strict adherence to moral values are considered a pre-requisite for mental health. Ayurveda aims to promote health, increase immunity and resistance-and to cure Disease.

Ayurveda understands that health is a reflection of when a person is living in harmony with nature and disease arises when a person is out of harmony with the cycles of nature. Ayurveda helps each individual realign their living patterns to bring about health and peace and to remember that their true nature is Spirit. Ayurveda gives equal importance to both preventive and curative aspects. Ayurveda offers methods of finding out the early stages of diseases that are still undetectable by the modern medical investigation. It is the knowledge of life in its entirety, that is body, mind, and soul.

The Ayurveda treatments can be classified into(Six):

- Massages.
- Dhara.
- Kizhi.
- Vasthi.
- Eye treatments.
- Panchakarma.

AYURVEDA HELP IN TACKLING MODERN DAY PROBLEMS

Stress has become a part of our daily lives. And everyday problems and situations bring stress in our life. Stress can be a result of fatigue and irritation and it can cause situations like pressure, loss of control, conflict, and uncertainty. Stress can happen from many situations and circumstances of life. Financial problems, unhappy relationships, work problems, and many other factors can leave a person in stress. When a person is stressed out his body creates extra energy to fight that stress. And thus it also creates an imbalance in the system.

Stress not only affects the mind but it affects the body as well. Stress is a natural part of anyone's life but an excessive amount of stress can result in hypertension and other diseases and ailments.

Ayurveda has its origin in India and it dates back to 5000 years or even more. It is a holistic healing system that not only helps to rejuvenate the body but also keeps a peaceful mind. According to

Ayurveda the body and mind should always be at peace and harmony with nature. The medicines, diet, lifestyle which are used and prescribed in Ayurveda are all-natural. Ayurveda healing and treatment depends mainly on the natural influences on our lives. The five natural elements and the six seasons play an important role in Ayurveda. The three doshas in the human body also depend on the natural elements of the environment. An imbalance within these doshas causes the body to function improperly.

Ayurveda believes in a healthy and harmonious lifestyle by nature. Ayurveda is a great stress reliever. And because of its immense success as the natural therapy for relieving stress and rejuvenating life it has become extremely popular in the western countries as well. People from the western countries who are always at constant stress and problems arising from the various spheres of life are finding solace and harmony in the Ayurveda treatments and therapies.

Ayurveda is a successful way of relieving stress and various natural therapies and treatments are applied to the patients to help restore a cured and peaceful mind and body. Ayurveda massages have gained enormous popularity in the western world. Various types of oil massages help to relieve stress. Some of the most popular massages and natural therapies include Kati Vasti useful for back pain and spinal cord injuries, Udwartanam useful for weight management, Shirodhara which highly effective for relieving of hypertension, mental disorders, headaches and stresses,

Pizhichil done for nervous disorders, rheumatic complaints, joint pain, and sexual weakness and Panchakarma which do the Panchakarma therapies to remove the various diseases from the body, and also remove the toxins from the body permanently.

Apart from the massages and therapies, there are various kinds of Ayurvedic herbal medicines which also help in beating the stress of everyday life. These medicines are available over the counter or in the Ayurveda centers where the treatments are given. People who are suffering from excessive stress may consult an Ayurveda physician for the treatment of stress and fatigue.

CHAPTER 4: AYURVEDA AND LIFE

HOW AYURVEDA HELPS YOUR LIFE

Ayurveda means the "science of life". It originated in India more than 10,000 years ago and is believed to be the oldest healing science in existence, from which all other systems emerged. Pronounced "Aa-your-vay-da", this ancient healing system has three **main focuses:**
- Healing illness
- Prevention of disease
- Longevity or age reversal

Laws of Nature and Spirituality, In essence, Ayurveda explains the laws of nature that cause health or disease. The first cause of the illness is said to be the loss of faith in the Divine or experiencing a spiritual emptiness. From here illness develops due to internal conditions (e.g., foods and li**q**uids) or external conditions (e.g., seasons, lifestyle). The main factors that cause poor health (also described as imbalance) are
- Poor digestion
- Weak immune systems.

When food is not properly digested it sits in the body. Nutrients are not absorbed and the food decays and forms toxins. These toxins cause most diseases in the body. Therefore, it is important to have good digestion.

The immune system can become depleted by poor nutrition, overwork, drugs, and other excesses. The finest essence of nutrition develops a life sap that protects the immune system, much like the sap of a tree heals the bruises in its bark. In addition to promoting physical health, it is the life sap that becomes transformed through meditation to produce mental peace and spiritual development. With all the immune disorders that are prevalent these days, it is even more important that persons develop their immune sap.

What Makes Ayurveda So Unique?
This spiritual science offers numerous unique benefits:
* It looks at people as individuals, not as a generic group.
* It heals from the root-cause of an illness, not merely treating the symptoms.
* Only natural therapies are offered.
* No side effects develop from the therapies.
* Therapies are inexpensive and effective

HOW DOES AYURVEDA WORK?

Tridosha Theory: The basic view of Ayurveda is that all of life (people, food, animals, nature, the universe, and diseases) are combinations of three energy-elements: air (called Vayu or Vata), fire (called Pitta), and water (called Kapha). When these elements are balanced, one is healthy. Illness is defined as an imbalance of these elements; all disorders are excesses of one or more elements.

People and the Elements: A person's constitution (dosha) is predominantly one or more of these elements. Each element relates to certain body types, foods and health concerns. By nature, whatever a person's constitution is, they tend for it to become excessed. For example, an air constitution person (Vayu dosha) is thin and bony. Physical symptoms of excess air include dry skin, cracking bones, gas, and constipation. Mental symptoms of excess air include fear, worry, anxiety, and nervousness. When an air constitution (Vayu dosha) person is balanced they are creative, adaptable and have no physical health concerns.

Ayurveda notes that certain foods increase air and other foods reduce air. In general, excess air is reduced by eating cooked or steamed foods and eating every three or four hours. Foods like carrots, rice, and mung beans reduce excess air. Broccoli, baked beans and barley increase air (e.g., they cause gas). Excessive lifestyles also increase the air element. Fire constitution people (Pitta dosha) tend towards excess heat. When healthy they are strong, make good leaders and are warm and goal-oriented. When the Pitta dosha is imbalanced, mentally they become hot-tempered, impatient, irritable.

Physically they develop heat-related disorders such as acne, rashes, diarrhea, ulcers, toxic blood, liver, kidney, gall bladder, heart and spleen disorders. Water constitutions (Kapha doshas) tend toward excess water. When healthy they are strong, muscular, calm and loyal. When water becomes excessed, they develop lethargy, and a hoarding or greedy nature. Physically they develop congestion, overweight, edema, heart and kidney problems, etc.

Health means balance. Each constitution has a natural tendency to become imbalanced or excessed. By eating foods and living a lifestyle that reduces the excesses, one remains balanced. Balancing produces healing, prevention, and reverses the aging process.

Many people have two or even all three elements in their constitution. In these cases, both elements tend toward excess. Thus foods and lifestyles that reduce both elements need to be followed.

WHAT THERAPIES DOES AYURVEDA OFFER?

Using a holistic approach, Ayurveda offers therapies for each of the five senses because different people learn better through different senses. Therapies include;
- Taste: Herbs and nutrition.
- Touch: Massage (abhyanga), Yoga, exercise.
- Smell: Aromatherapy.
- Sight: Color therapy.
- Hearing: Music therapy, mantra meditation, chanting. Spiritual therapies include meditation, living ethically, and working in a career that one loves or is purposeful.

Environmental factors are also considered from this holistic outlook. These therapies include house, apartment, and office structure and astrological effects. These are sciences unto themselves. Vedic architecture (Vastu Shastra) and Chinese Feng Shui (pronounced Fung sh way) deal with the laws of nature that integrate the earth, the person and the planets and stars. The exterior and interior design of buildings can also enhance balance or cause imbalance. Vedic astrology (Jyotish) is the science of understanding the laws of nature of the planets and stars, and how they influence us.

What Does Holistic Mean?
Holistic has two meanings.
- It looks at the whole of one's life. Health and disease are byproducts of all aspects of one's life: nutrition, career, mental frame, family and social activities and spiritual life. If one area is weakened, all areas begin to suffer. If a person is unhappy at work, it will affect all other areas of life.
- Holistic means are holy. Ayurveda reminds us that to have and maintain true health, one needs to take some quiet time for spiritual development. The goal of life is Self-Realization. This is a state of unshakable Divine mental peace.

AGE GRACEFULLY THROUGH AYURVEDA

Ayurveda is the traditional medical system of India. The word Ayurveda comes from two Sanskrit words viz - AYU=life and VEDA=knowledge. So the literal meaning of Ayurveda means 'knowledge about life' or in a broad sense, knowledge of perfect living. This concept of life that one is becoming free from all ailments and death sows the seeds for the development of geriatric science which evolved as one of the eight branches of Ayurveda.

Ancient saints of India developed Ayurveda by aiming in two aspects. They are prevention of disease by enjoying optimum health and cure the disease by living harmoniously with nature. Geriatric treatment in Ayurveda revolves around the old age ailments to delay and prevent the aging process, prevent complications of existing diseases, reducing wear and tear of tissues. Chronology of aging in Ayurveda is Childhood, Development, Complexion, Intellectual grasping power, Skin health, Visual acuity, Sexual excellence, Vigor, Intellect, Manual activities, Response to stimulus, Life. These factors are decaying in each decade. So death will occur at 120 years. In comparison with today's life status, it can be understood that we should adopt the ways of ayurvedic living for optimum health so that we can live up to 120 years gracefully without any diseases.

Irrespective of one's chronological age Ayurveda looks at the quality of these bodily factors. Accordingly, his body age is calculated. If one loses visual acuity (presbyopia) at 40 years, Ayurveda calculates his age as 60 years irrespective of his chronological age. Ayurveda has three main domains of therapeutic regimens which are the powerful tools to address the issues of aging. They are known as Rasayana therapy [RT] (Chiefly rejuvenative), vajeekarana therapy [VT] (chiefly Aphrodisiac) and yoga therapy (chiefly meditation techniques).

RT consists of the use of some specific herbal medicine formulations which are being used uniquely. These therapies were used by ancient scholars for the Prevention of aging physiology by several means. RT enhances the health of the brain, heart and blood vessels and bones. RT is highly neurotonic and these formulations are found to be the richest source of free radical scavengers and fight against reactive oxygen species production in our body. The following drugs are examples of RT drugs. Emblica Officinalis, Tinospora cordifolia, Tribulus Terrestris, Asparagus racemosa, etc.

VT is a branch of Ayurveda is dealing with the sexual excellence of one individual. These are also consisting of a good number of herbal formulations which are found to be effective in increasing testicular blood circulation, maintain testosterone level optimally in the blood, and prevent the wear and tear and senile atrophic changes of the genital organs. Withania somnifera, Ipomea batatus, Mucuna prurita are examples of aphrodisiac drugs used in Ayurveda. They are also found to be the richest source of phytoestrogens and Phyto testosterone.

These ayurvedic herbal drugs don't contain any heavy metals or any other toxic materials. So they can be used effectively even for a long time. But there is the usage of several mineral drugs in Ayurveda and they are not having above mentioned rejuvenative or aphrodisiac property mostly. They have to be used strictly with proper medical advice.

Yoga therapy is the concept of health in terms of physical, mental and spiritual well-being date back to the origin of Ayurveda. So sufficient emphasis had been given to the yoga techniques to maintain and restore physical, mental and spiritual health during old age too. So ancient saints of India writes as the mental well being is the most rejuvenating drug in the world. This yoga technique harmonizes the psycho neuro endocrinal functions, psycho neuroimmunological functions. Facing senescence through a combination of RT, VT and yoga techniques will be certainly grateful to attain the physical, mental and spiritual well being of an individual. Indians consider this approach as a boon from their Ayurveda to age gracefully and to combat the problems of senescence.

CHAPTER 5: AYURVEDA POWER

THE UNIQUE POWER OF AYURVEDA TO HEAL ANY HEALTH PROBLEM

What comes to our mind if we think about any type of treatment? It will be allopathy or homeopathy. No wonder that Ayurveda secures no position in the list of the trustworthiness in the mind of many people. This Ayurveda has some kind of power that will go deep inside or in the root to eradicate any disease. This medication, from ancient times, is somehow overlooked or ignored by the users. The Ayurvedic Medicines exist or not we rarely bother! Things will get changed once you start believing it.

Ayurveda works if someone trusts

The young generation tends to give a stare to these age-old medicines. They consider this type of medicine belongs to the pre-historic era. Ayurvedic treatment needs patience as well as time. All those who are in a hurry; this type of medicine will not be good for them. You can rely on Ayurveda if you enough time to use it regularly, without making any kind of mistakes. These Ayurvedic Medicines have no side effects. Yes, because of the main ingredients of this medicine or herbs. Taste-wise it will not be great of course. There are so many people who all have shown their faith in Ayurveda and got the desired result. You can be one of them easily. The biggest benefit of this Ayurveda is that it is not costly. Any and every kind of health-related problems can easily be resolved by the touch of Ayurveda.

Why should you switch over to Ayurveda?

- A non-curable disease like Cancer and all can be cured by the power of herbs.
- Those who all are afraid of operations will be the greatest option for them. Ayurveda believes that surgery is the last step.
- Chronic diseases can easily get cured by Ayurveda medicines.
- These medicines are free from chemicals. That means no worry of side effects at all.
- Consumption of these types of medicines will cure the problem as well as develop the overall health condition by increasing the rate of metabolism, decrease the level of stress and bring back the obstinacy back into your life.
- These types of medicines will go to the root to eradicate the problem. That means that a particular person will not suffer from the same problem again.

Availability of these Ayurveda medicine ayurvedic Medicines Manufacturers and dealers must be there in your locality also. Why don't you visit one of those medicine shops and read out the compositions of these medicines by yourself to kick away all misconceptions regarding Ayurveda and its result? At that time only you will start believing in the magic of Ayurveda.

7 BENEFICIAL AYURVEDA SPICES

Would you like your family to bond and have wonderful, magical times together? How would you like to have your children happier, calmer, better behaved, and more appreciative? Would you like to reduce the need to take your children to the doctor as often as you do? Imagine that your family's health issues naturally clear up; would you like to live this way?

Welcome back to the idea of 'Cooking', and specifically, 'Ayurvedic Cooking'!

There are many benefits from doing things on your own, including making your own simple, home-cooked meals from scratch. Buying fresh fruits, vegetables, and whole grains and beans save you loads of money compared to eating out and increases health and happiness (from being healthy). Cooking together brings the family together; simple, delicious, and healthful meals can be made within half an hour; and overall health noticeably improves (eg, often allergies and other illnesses improve). Each benefit is exciting enough to merit its discussion. In this article, we will focus on 7 easily available cooking improve the taste of the foods and can be used to improve health. Many of the ways these address common health issues have been shown through scientific research.

Ayurveda offers your family a more personal insight and use of the herbs, helping you choose which herbs are most suited to your constitution or dosha. Thus foods can be delicious as well as healthful for your particular palette. If you need to know your dosha, free online dosha tests are available.

What makes these seemingly insignificant and oft-overlooked spices such powerful allies is that they improve the digestion. Ayurveda notes that the cause of most physical illnesses is due to poor digestion; well-digested foods mean nutrition is absorbed and fed to the body for health and immune strength. So let's take a more grateful look at these 'sacred crumbs'

•Black Pepper

Best for Dosha: Vayu and Kapha dosha (constitution) people

Best for Conditions: Burns up ama very well, colds, flu, cough, gargle for sore throat, fevers, colon cleanse, digests fat and obesity; metabolism, mucus, expectorant, sinus congestion, cold extremities, raises Agni, epileptic seizures, with honey, clear Kapha from the system in the morning. External-inflammations, urticaria, erysipelas.

•Cumin

Best for Dosha: All

Best for Conditions: digests bread, along with caraway, fennel and dill relatives; colitis, gas, digestion, abdominal pain, distention, for overeating and eating heavy foods.

*Cardamom

Best for Dosha: All
Best for Conditions: Absorption of nutrients, asthma, bronchitis, colds, cough, excellent for stomach complaints, hoarseness, indigestion, loss of taste, helps the spleen and pancreas, reduces Kapha in lungs and stomach, stimulates the mind, with milk it reduces mucus formation, detoxifies caffeine in coffee, nervous digestion, vomiting, headache, belching, acid indigestion, nausea, expels Vayu in colon and digests foods in colon, convalescing from diarrhea, biliousness, respiratory disorders, involuntary urination.
Spiritual Uses: spiritual peace and purity; gives clarity and joy
Antidote: Helps digest foods if they create sluggish digestion. Ice cream, milk, cold or sweet foods like bananas, coffee

*Coriander

Best for Dosha: All
Best for Conditions: Griping, flatulent colic, rheumatism, neuralgia, indigestion, vomiting, intestinal disorders, removes excess Kapha, eyewash, conjunctivitis, relieves internal heat and thirst, skin/rash problems, urogenital system

(burning urethra, cystitis, infections, etc.), sore throat, allergies, hay fever, for all Pitta disorders, burning, juice for allergies, hay fever, and skin rashes (and externally as well); antidotes hot pungent foods, bleeding hemorrhoids. Used to balance very hot foods and spices (eg, chilies).

• Fennel

Best for Dosha: All
Best for Conditions: Abdominal pain (gas or indigestion), menstrual cramps, hernia, diarrhea, colic, vomiting, morning sickness, nausea, anorexia, cough, dry cough, promotes semen, increases vision, raises Agni, difficult or burning urination, digestion-children and elderly; promotes menstruation, nursing mothers-increases breast milk flow.

• Fenugreek

Best for Dosha: Vayu & Kapha
Best for Conditions: Longevity, nerves, allergies, arthritis, skin, rejuvenation, diabetes, allergies, bronchitis, flu, chronic cough, dysentery, dyspepsia, convalescence, edema, toothache, sciatica, neurasthenia, counters cold (i.e., extremities, abdominal pain, indigestion, respiratory and reproductive systems, hair growth, promotes breast milk flow, liver hypo-function, seminal debility, debility, outdoor winter work). Precaution: Do not use when pregnant.

·Turmeric

Best for Dosha: Kapha/ good for all doshas in moderation

Best for Condition: Amenorrhea, anemia, arthritis, blood purifier, blood tissue formation, circulation, cooking spice, cough, diabetes, worms, jaundice, eye problems, fevers, gas, hemorrhoids, edema, indigestion, ligament stretching, metabolism regulator; mucus relief, and hysteria (from inhaling fumes); pharyngitis, protein-digesting, skin disorders, abscess, urinary diseases, wound, and bruise healer; a natural antibiotic that also improves intestinal flora; inflammatory bowel syndrome (e.g., ulcerative colitis), Chron's Disease, chronic hepatitis, chronic bronchial asthma, psoriasis, all inflammatory conditions.

Spiritual Uses: Gives one the Divine Goddess's energy and prosperity; Chakra and subtle body cleanser; limber for Yoga asana practice

Precautions: Do not use if pregnant, with excess Pitta, with acute jaundice or hepatitis.

So bring the family into the kitchen and share the magic of cooking, sprinkle a little more love in your life; save money, enhance health, and discover just how sacred the cooking experience can be!

CHAPTER 6: AYURVEDA UNTYPICAL TYPES AND SEX

AYURVEDA - UNTYPICAL TYPES

Among ancient Eastern methods, which medicine and the beauty industry turns to more and more, Ayurveda is the leader. This isn't just fashion or exotic trends. In the five thousand years that Ayurveda has existed, it has proved to be a serious science, which can do such things that often, can not be done by official medicine.

There are whole tractates about Ayurveda, which are now available to the wide audience. Therefore, we will only go over some underlying aspects, which demonstrate the modernity and timeliness of Ayurvedic teachings. If we look at Ayurveda outside of the philosophical environment and very ancient context, it is simply teachings about the healthy way of life - "the science of life". Ayurveda tells us that the length and quality of life depend on the person; what he eats, how he behaves, and what efforts he takes on the way to perfection of body, mind, and spirit.

Ayurveda offers a whole set of methods, which can help successfully progress on this path. All the doctors - experts in the sphere of Ayurvedic knowledge – say that their knowledge roots from the first teacher, Charaka Samhita, who wrote the guide to Ayurveda. After receiving this knowledge from sages, who have granted him the ability to give amrita (the nectar of immortality), Charaka gave them book format, and thus was the first author of Ayurvedic texts. The chain of teaching the next generations of doctors began with him.

Untypical Types
Any treatment is proscribed with the consideration of prakri (the patient's constitution). According to Ayurveda, all people are divided into certain types. For example, muscular people with red hair, who are inclined to become irritated and even aggressive, belong to the category of pure Pitta people. The Kapha types are massive people with thick skin. They are slow and sleepy and usually strive to collect material riches. Vatta, on the contrary, is thin people with dry hair. They have weak joints and are usually inclined to be scared and to worry. There is a whole set of signs – not only constitutional but also inner and psychological signs, - which can determine which type a person belongs to. There are many formal methods; it is enough to fill in a form to find out which qualities a person possesses. However, this does not mean that Ayurveda strictly divides people into only three types.

There are combined, "dual" types, and besides that, there are different amounts of righteousness, passion, and ignorance in each type. A certain diet, exercises, methods of cleaning and rejuvenating the organism, a special set of spices, herbs, and preparations are recommended for each type. The ability of Ayurvedic doctors depends on how well they can determine the methods of treatment and improving the health of each person. They also have to give recommendations about the way of life, advise herbs and spices, oils and types of massage, which harmonize the mind and emotions, colors and precious stones, yoga and meditation exercises for every patient.

WOMAN AND CHILDCARE IN AYURVEDA

Ayurvedic women and childcare rules layout solid action plans to ensure the health of women and children. In India, women have ascribed divinity, solely because of their ability to give birth to a child and thereby retaining the human race on the face of the earth.
Bala chikitsa (child care) is the wing of Ayurveda that deals with women and childcare. Bala means a child and chikitsa means treatment. According to Ayurveda woman and children are no separate entities but inseparable factors. This is because the health of the woman during pregnancy directly affects the health of the baby. Any post-natal disease to mothers can also deprive the child of essential nutrients in the form of breast milk.

Ayurveda also considers women as the first teacher of a child and every aspect of the proper development of a child is directly linked to the physical and mental health of the mother.

Woman and childcare in Ayurveda in principle starts before the formation of the fetus inside the womb. Healthy fetus formation is the result of the union of a healthy man and a healthy woman, at the right time and in the right manner.

This branch of Ayurveda deals with impotence, infertility, prenatal, natal and postnatal care. Neonatal care has significant importance according to Ayurvedic concepts. The care given to a newborn child is equivalent to a lifetime of health care. The right treatments and care given to a newborn baby at the right times will ensure the healthy development of the child as a person and contributing member to society.

The basis of a woman and child care Ayurveda is found in ancient Ayurvedic treatises - Ashtanga Hridaya, Sushrutha Samhita, Charaka Samhita, and Vagbhata Samhita.

Vagbhata Samhitha and Ashtanga Hridaya (both by Acharya Vagbhata) has comprehensive guidelines about day to daycare of a pregnant woman and a newborn child. Both mental and physical health of a mother is important to the progeny. There are specified treatment and caring methods for expecting women in Ayurvedic women and child care.

This includes a highly nutritive diet specially formulated for each month of development of the fetus and diet that ensures lactation. Specific issues like nausea, vomiting, constipation, etc that occurs during the pregnancy have effective treatments in Ayurveda woman and child care.

The food and medicines also prepare the woman for the smooth delivery of a healthy baby.

The food items that an expecting or nursing mother takes must be pure and free from any toxins like pesticides or chemicals. Any violation from the Ayurvedic rules can lead to the birth of an unhealthy child.

AYURVEDA AND SEX

Sex, according to Ayurveda and according to Ayurveda and the Vedas, is a divine process that is responsible for the very existence of the human race on the face of the earth. Kamasutra, the ancient science of love and lovemaking describes in detail a variety of factors involved in practicing safe and fulfilling sex.

In India, sex was never considered something to shun about. According to Ayurveda, a child is an asset. From having intercourse to delivering children and bringing them up with a healthy body, mind and imparting in them, the training to see life in a positive life and showing them the good way of life is an elaborate process. One noticeable thing about Ayurveda is the relative silence about family planning, contraception methods, or abortion - why destroy the greatest asset one can get? Sal-Santanangal (or children of good qualities, physically, mentally and spiritually) is the ultimate aim of sex.

Vageekarana Chikitsa (Aphrodisiac Treatment)

Aphrodisiac therapy or treatment has a prominent place in Ayurveda. It is part of Vrisha, one anga or branch in ashtanga or eight principle branches of Ayurveda. Removing the imbalances of doshas or tridosha (Vata, pitta, Kapha) comes before vageekarana chikitsa (aphrodisiac therapy).

Good physical qualities, semen quantity, and quality is the aim of vajeekarana chikitsa.

There is also a list of qualifications for both men and women. The man should be compatible with his woman in physical, mental, and on an astrological basis. A man shall go to his wife only. Meeting other women is strictly prohibited in Ayurveda. The only place to ejaculate semen is vagina - masturbation and all other forms of unnatural sex are prohibited.

Although Kamasutra suggests 64 different sexual positions, Ayurveda recognizes only the common method -woman bottom and man top. Experimenting on this for bodily pleasure causes a woman's body to a position in different forms, which can cause immediately long-term faults to a woman's body and also to the child. Vageekarana chikitsa or Jaara chikitsa (aphrodisiac therapy) suggests Panchakarma for purification of physiology and semen. Panchakarma is not necessary for women because of physical peculiarities.

Ayurveda suggests a physical union of loving couples as the one way to enjoy divine pleasure. Here an assembly of panchendriya (Five Senses - touch, sight, etc.), physical organs, and mind take place.

AYURVEDA AND PREMATURE EJACULATION

The practitioners of modern Ayurveda claim that a male individual experiences premature ejaculation when the suitable balance of the Vata dosha in his body has been upset, causing disruptions in nerve impulses, circulation, and respiration, which in turn leads to a very quick excretion of Shukra (semen) during sex.

In an attempt to restore the balance and, in turn, cure PE, several medicinal preparations are used. Herbs like the Himalayan shilajit and dhatupaustic churna and other assorted substances are used in an attempt to improve sexual prowess by maintaining a healthy balance between mind and body.

As for the question of whether these preparations work to cure PE, it's not an easy one to answer. Such treatments, for example, don't have any clinical trials and there're therefore no statistical data to back up the claims of those advocating Ayurveda.

There are obvious patterns between the wisdom of the ancient East and the scientific medicine of the modern West that are in agreement here.

It is not difficult, for example, to see that the disruptions of the Vata dosha in Ayurveda are very similar to a phenomenon we'd refer to as "stress" (which is a well known contributing factor to PE) here in the West, or that Ayurveda's focus on "exercises" and yoga strike a close resemblance to the sort of exercises and mental healing you'd get in sexual therapy and psychotherapy sessions for PE treatment.

What's in the ancient East as non-scientific wisdom has long since been refined and made safer in the West. But for us in the West, there's something very exotic about such alternative medicines from ancient times I suppose. Perhaps this is part of the reason why we find these treatment approaches appealing still even though, when all is said and done, they offer nothing profoundly different from what's already available here at home, made safer and better no less.

With safety concerns having already been raised about Ayurveda by two U.S. studies, finding about 20% of Ayurvedic treatments containing toxic levels of heavy metals such as lead, mercury and arsenic, and concerns over the use of herbs that contain toxic compounds and the lack of quality control in Ayurvedic facilities, I argue that our love affair with the exotic in this case is not only unnecessary but also downright dangerous.

CHAPTER 7: YOGA AND AYURVEDA

YOGA AYURVEDA - AN INTRODUCTION TO UNDERSTANDING THE BODY-MIND-SPIRIT CONNECTION WITH YOGA AYURVEDA

Ayurveda is an ancient Indian healing system that allows you to gain insight into your body's mind. It explains how to keep the body-mind balanced with the internal and external environment, and functioning optimally.

When you have insight into your unique body-mind nature, you understand:
- What your potential is
- Your likes and dislikes
- Why you do the things you do
- How you are likely to respond to stress
- What diseases you are more likely to succumb to
- What your dominant tendencies are, both negative and positive

The ancient seers realized that the 5 universal elements exist within all of creation. That the qualities or metaphors of earth, water, fire, air, and ether is present within nature in various combinations. For example: observe the proportion of solidness - earth - that's within a palm tree and an oak; the quality of lightness -

fire - within garlic and pepper; and the quality of movement - air - within a tortoise and a hare.

A unique combination of the elements, called doshas, form the body, and each body must care for it its distinctive way to achieve and maintain balance with the environment. This is essential for health as an excess or deficiency of an element can ultimately result in disease.

BODY MIND SPIRIT AND YOGA THERAPY

In the Yoga Ayurveda connection, Ayurveda emphasizes cleansing and building the physical body through herbs, massage, diet, and lifestyle, and recommends yoga, meditation and breathing techniques for healing body mind spirit. With an understanding of your body-mind nature, you'll be alert to override the natural tendency to select those yoga exercises, meditation, and breathing techniques that create imbalance.

Yoga therapy with Ayurveda would be guided by the principles of Ayurveda. Ayurveda recognizes the cycles of time and season and their effect on the body. The six different times of each day affect the doshas, and therefore each body. Each season of the year will increase one or two doshas within the body. And this ancient Indian healing system acknowledges three different times of our lives that also affect the body and mind.

In the body mind spirit connection, the mind changes constantly. Cool and calm one moment, then agitated another and feeling dull and lethargic yet another time. And when we understand our predisposition to a specific emotion like fear, anger or greed, these enemies of the spirit can be tackled.

Yoga therapy and Ayurveda can rejuvenate your body and bring compassion and understanding to relationships. Get to know your body-mind nature and understand why you do the things you do.

YOGA AND AYURVEDIC TREATMENTS - A CORRELATION BETWEEN MIND AND BODY

As the world is developing in technology day by day we are moving away from nature. We have depleted nature's every gift, polluted the environment with deforestation. Nature is reacting to us in the form of natural calamities and certain diseases. Moreover, in this fast pace life, we don't allow our body to fight with any illness and take man-made drugs forgetting that the same nature has a cure for all disturbances. In such adverse circumstances, yoga and Ayurveda still show hope to be connected with nature. This provides treatment for almost all diseases.

Yoga and ayurvedic treatments have a different

approach that works not only on illness but tries to find out the root cause thus eliminating it permanently. Yoga is very effective in stabilizing nervous disorders, stress, constipation, reducing anxiety and depression, eliminating fatigue and even helpful in diseases like cancer and aids. Yoga treatments include a no. of exercises, asana, chanting of mantras, meditation, etc. Ayurvedic treatments involve massage, ayurvedic face rejuvenation, Shirodhara, and various other oil treatments.

Different postures during yoga include sitting, standing or lying down to relax your muscles and other body parts. Meditation is the most effective way to reduce stress. Here equilibrium is established between mind and body and gradually your mind becomes so free that you feel to be present there only physically and mind roams in the universe. This gives you great relaxation and makes you feel active. Different asana during yoga fills you with different energy and power.

While in ayurvedic treatments, toxic substances from the body are reduced or removed through various ayurvedic remedies. These remedies are prepared from using a variety of herbs, minerals, and sometimes a few animal products also. Ayurveda believes that the body is made of Vata, Pitta, and Kapha. Any imbalance in these three is the main cause of diseases in an individual, so ayurvedic treatments always try to bring them in harmony. Ayurveda not only keeps you healthy but also beautiful and attractive by making your skin healthy, shiny and glow.

Many people believe that yoga treatment just includes a few exercises that you can do yourself and can be healthy. But it's not so, there are various technical approaches to adopt yoga therapy. If you adopt it home without any instructions then be careful because one wrong move can make you still for a lifetime. If not a yoga instructor, you can consider the internet, books and any other sources. Moreover, yoga is not the solution to all the diseases. Though a mastered yogic can find a remedy for any said diseases you should not try yoga for any diseases without any consultations.

Yoga and ayurvedic treatments are prevalent from ancient times. But these days they have to gain more popularity and various yoga and ayurvedic centers have been established not only in India but also in foreign countries. There are more foreigners than Indians to follow such techniques in curing their illness.

ENHANCE YOUR OVERALL PERSONALITY WITH AYURVEDA & YOGA

Ayurveda, literally meaning 'the Science of Life', shares an age-old relationship with India. Ayurveda and Yoga are evolved from India only and have been practiced here for centuries. It is a holistic healing science in which the medicines are prepared from natural and organic materials making it the only eco-friendly medical science now known.

The origin of this ancient Indian medical science dates back to the era when Vedas (the oldest available classics of the world) was created. This system of traditional medicine native to India deals with the maintenance of health and relief from disease. It focuses on exercise, yoga, meditation, and massage.

Basic Principles

Ayurveda says that the human body consists of three primary life forces or biological humor (Tridoshas)- Vatha, Pitha, and Kapha. Proper health requires a balance among these three life forces. Otherwise, these can cause a state of unhealthiness or disease. The Ayurvedic treatment is known for its 'Panchakarma therapy', which includes cleaning enemas, nasal medication, Purgation, Emesis, and bloodletting. There are a total of eight disciplines of Ayurveda treatment, namely:

- Shalya-chikitsa (Surgery)
- Salakyam (Treatment of diseases above the clavicle)
- Kaaya-chikitsa (Internal medicine)
- Bhuta Vidya (Demonic possession)
- Kaumarabhrtyam (Paediatrics)
- Agadatantram (Toxicology)
- Rasayanam (Prevention and building immunity)
- Vajikaranam (Aphrodisiacs)

Ayurvedic TreatmentsAyurvedic therapies work

on the processes of 'Tonification' and 'Reduction'. On one hand, Tonification methods nurture insufficiency in the body while Reduction therapies, on the other, decrease excesses in the body. Reduction therapies are further categorized as 'Pacification' (done with herbs, fasting, exercise, sunbathing and exposure to wind) and 'Purification' (a special form of therapy for elimination of the disease-causing humor).

Ayurveda tours in India offer hundreds of Ayurveda therapies specially designed for different kinds of disorders/diseases. A few most popular therapies are Pizhichil, Njavarkizhi, Sirodhara, Vasthi, Sirovasthi, Nasyam, Kizhi, Dhara, Avisnanam, etc.

Ayurveda is practiced in various Ayurveda Resorts in different parts of India, out of which Kerala and a few regions in north India top the chart. The equable climate and natural abundance of forests (herbs and medicinal plants) in Kerala make it the best-suited place for Ayurvedic treatments. Kerala is believed to be the only state in India which practices this system of medicine with complete dedication.

AYURVEDA AS A WAY OF LIFE

Ayurveda is a popular and traditional natural healing system in India. It involves some simple practical guidelines for leading a healthy and stress-free life. It involves certain practices that will bring the perfect physical and mental balance. Ayurveda essentially means the science of life and it teaches man to live in harmony with nature to achieve good health.

As every person has a different constitution Ayurveda seeks to balance the doshas or humor in a person which is the basis of good health. Ayurveda is a holistic system of medicine and seeks to prevent as well as cure diseases. It tries to cure diseases in the mental, physical and spiritual levels and in that way is gaining recognition the world over as a good alternative system of medicine.

The three important principles which govern the normal functioning of the human body according to Ayurveda are Vata, Pitta, and Kapha. They symbolize the three bhutas namely air, fire, and water. Any disequilibrium in the three doshas will lead to an imbalance in the body in some form that in turn leads to diseases. Ayurveda encompasses eight branches of treatment ranging from surgery, internal medicine, childhood diseases, toxicology, psychiatry, and many more disciplines.

There are also weight loss packages and traditional panchakarma treatments offered at the ayurvedic centers which aim a host of diseases including depression, chronic headache, and other stress-related disorders. The panchakarma treatment also helps in detoxifying, rejuvenating and balancing both mind and body. Ayurveda also gives advice on food and lifestyle changes to be incorporated into one's life that will kick start all-round health. Its popularity lies in the fact that it combines both preventive and curative aspects of medicine in treating ailments of different kinds.

AYURVEDA AND YOGA

Those, who think that just by practicing a set of difficult physical exercises, they achieve a state of enlightenment, are deeply mistaken. Working with the body is only the first step on the way to spiritual progress. When one controls the functions of one's organism, he prepares himself for the transformation of the soul.

Ayurveda is connected to yoga. But, not that yoga, which seems to be a set of strange poses and exercises. In reality, yoga isn't just physical exercises, it requires spiritual progress. In Hindi, yoga means "connection", which directs our mind in the right direction and control our emotions.

Those, who think that just by practicing a set of difficult physical exercises, they achieve a state of enlightenment, are deeply mistaken. Working with the body is only the first step on the way to spiritual progress. When one controls the functions of one's organism, he prepares himself for the transformation of the soul.

Yoga is only a part of Ayurveda, one of the steps to achieving a righteous way of life. Practicing only yoga will give results and will have a good effect on the organism, but the meaning of "lifestyle" is a lot wider. A set of physical exercises, meditation exercises, aromatherapy, diagnostics by the pulse, Ayurvedic recipes, individual mineral additives, and other food additives – all these are bricks of a beautiful and slender building, which we know as Ayurveda.

YOGA - THE PERFECT WAY TO PERFECT HEALTH

The regular practice of yoga provides us with immunity against all diseases. Lakhs of People in the west have appreciated the benefits of yoga and are now regular practitioners of this form due to the benefits it brings. Though yoga was an offshoot of Hindu philosophy and was intended to bring human beings in union with the creator, it has now been practiced primarily to improve the physical and mental health of an individual. Yoga Sutra, written 2000 years ago by Patanjali, provides us with the earliest and the most authentic treatise on yoga. He dwelt at length on all aspects of yoga and has also described the eight stages of yoga discipline.

Eight principles
- Yamas- Restraints
- Niyamas- Observance of austerity, purity, contentment, study, surrender of ego.
- Asanas- Physical postures or exercises.
- Pranayama- Breathing control.
- Partyahara- Withdrawal of the senses.
- Dharana- Concentration of the mind.
- Dhyana- Meditation.
- Samadhi- Attainment of the superconscious state.

Rules and Regulations

As yoga is a time tested and proven scientific system meant for physical, spiritual and mental excellence, certain rules and regulations are to be followed for successful results.

- Though there is no specific time for doing yoga, morning is the best time to perform yoga. One should then stick to this time regularly and should practice regularly for 15 minutes each day, 5 days a week.
- The place where one practices yoga alone should be neat, clean and airy.
- Yoga should as far as possible be practiced on an empty stomach. In case one has consumed food, he should wait for at least 2 hours before practicing yoga. Hot and spicy foods, excess

intake of tea, coffee, alcohol, and drugs are best avoided.
- One should relax for 5 to 10 seconds between asanas.
- One should be neat and clean both in person and also in his dress and should neither be tired nor under physical stress.
- The mind should be free from worries, tension, and anxiety while practicing.
- Women should avoid practicing yoga during their menstrual periods and pregnant women should practice moderately.

Asanas are certain body postures that an individual takes in the course of performing yoga and these form an integral part of the yoga. These asanas are designed to promote the physical, spiritual and mental well being of an individual. There are several asanas and each one has a special name, form, offer particular benefits, and have a distinct way of performing. Asanas are highly beneficial and help to overhaul, rejuvenate and bring the entire body constitution into a state of equilibrium. We give below a few of the common asanas that are widely practiced in India.

- **Surya Namaskar.** This means greeting and bowing to the sun. This is the most widely practiced asana. And all asanas usually begin with greeting the sun. This form is useful in nourishing and energizing the upper part of the human body.
- **Uttham Pada Asana.** In this form of asana, one lifts the legs upwards. This posture is

particularly beneficial in strengthening the spinal cord.

- **Paschimothan Asana.** Also called the forward bend, this completely stretches the entire back of the body. Though a bit strenuous, this is a very helpful pose for the entire body right from the skull up to the heels.
- **Bhujanga Asana.** This is called the cobra pose and is done to give flexibility to the spine.
- **Salabha Asana-** This is known as the locust posture and helps strengthen and activate the lower part of the body from the waist downwards. And to derive maximum benefit from this posture, one should practice it after the cobra pose.
- **Sarvanga Asana.** This is considered as one of the most important of the asanas. In this posture, the weight of the entire body is made to rest on the shoulders. This also helps to stretch the neck and the upper back regions to the maximum.
- **Matsya Asana.** Also called the fish pose, this form helps to fill the lungs with air and improve the ability to float in water. It is recommended that this asana be performed after the sarvanga asana.
- **Dhanur Asana.** This pose helps to give a backward bend to the spine and all the muscles of the back from neck to the lower back. It is advised that dhanur asana be performed together with the locust pose.
- **Hala Asana.** This is called the plow pose. In this form, the person bends forward to the

maximum. This is highly useful in providing strength and flexibility to all parts of the back and neck.

- **Shava Asana.** This is called the corpse pose as the position adopted resembles the posture of a corpse. This is one of the most commonly practiced asanas and helps give relaxation to the body and mind.

Benefits

The regular practice of yoga provides immense benefits to all who practice it. Its wide acceptance throughout the world is a measure of its efficacy and the help it provides in improving the physical, mental and spiritual health of an individual. Yoga alters brain wave activities reflecting in increased relaxation and a better-focused mind. It is effective in preventing heart diseases. Yoga also helps lower blood pressure. It guards against insomnia and improves memory and strengthens the muscles. It brings in psychological changes that will reflect in the overall health and well being of an individual.

Yoga techniques are being increasingly used as a supplementary therapy for such diseases as cancer, diabetes, arthritis, asthma, etc. It helps to kick the habit of smoking. The modern world has much to gain from yoga. Yoga is the way and the means

YOGA AND PRIME AYURVEDIC TREATMENTS

Yoga is one of the most prized gifts to us from ancient India. Yoga comes from the Latin word 'Yuj' meaning 'to unite'. It is not just about physical postures, but it is, more importantly, a spiritual art that links one's consciousness with the universal consciousness. Certainly, we are always preoccupied with perceiving the outside world without giving time to the inner self. This ancient art gives you the secrets of finding inner peace and transcendence through the techniques of exercise, breathing, and meditation which are constantly evolving and innovating. Yoga that we see today in the modern world is an integrated version of ancient Yogic concepts with modern medical and psychological techniques.

Ayurveda is a Sanskrit word composed of two words 'Ayur' and 'Veda'. The former means life and the latter knowledge or science, together, it means the science of life. It is an ancient medical science which deals with the body, mind, and soul. This science does not only help in treating illness, but it also helps ensure for leading a long illness-free, healthy and happy life. Using natural plants as the source of making its medicines, it has become very reliable and popular among modern scholars of medical science around the globe. With this, the enthusiasm of inquisitiveness has aroused among them to know more about Ayurvedic knowledge.

Ayurveda treatments

Ayurveda treatments can be best described as the treatment of man as a whole. Ayurvedic medicines are mainly made from natural plants and their side-effects are almost none. Its treatment is based on the principles that enlightenment could be only achieved by those with good mental and physical health. Ayurveda uses different forms of treatments for various types of problems.

Some of the prime treatments of Ayurveda are:

•**Pizhichil:** In this kind of treatment, warmish herbal oil is applied throughout the body by two to four trained therapists in some special rhythmic way for about 60-90 minutes a day for 7-21 days. This treatment is for pain, dislocation, and tensions in joints and limbs. It is also for that person with paralysis and pregnant women with the problem of the absence of effective uterine contractions during labor. The treatment lasts from 14 to 28 days. Some people took this treatment for maintaining physical fitness against early aging. Hardening of body tissue can also be prevented by this treatment.

•**Njavarakizhi:** In this case, some medicinal puddings, in the form of boluses tied up in muslin bags, are externally applied to the body and made the body perspire. This type of treatment is mostly practiced in Kerala. It is mainly for all types of diseases of the nervous system, joints pain, chronic rheumatism, diseases caused by defects in blood. It helps in building a strong and solid body with good muscle system.

- **Dhara:** Here, certain herbal oils, medicated milk or buttermilk are poured on the forehead for about 45 minutes a day for 7-21 days. There are other subcategories for this treatment such as Thakradhara, Sthanyadhara, and Tailadhara. Thakradhara is for treating against premature graying of hair, headache, fatigue, diabetes, dislocated joints, weakness, tiredness, eye diseases, ear, throat and nose illnesses. Sthanyadhara is for treating extremely high fever especially among children and Tailadhara for sinuses, paralysis, and headache.
- **Vasthi:** Herbal oils or herbal extracts are applied through the rectum daily for 5-25 days. This treatment is meant for paralysis, hemiplegia, arthritis, numbness, gastric, frequent constipation and Rheumatism.
- **Sirovasthi:** In this process, specific lukewarm herbal oils are poured into the cap fitted on the head and kept it for about 15-60 minutes per day according to the condition of the patients. This treatment is for loss of tactile sensation, facial paralysis, dryness of mouth, throat, and nostrils, chronic headache and other vatha related diseases.
- **Udvarthanam:** In this treatment, the body is massaged with certain herbal powder for about 30 minutes for 14-28 days. This treatment is for diseases like hemiplegia, paralysis, typical rheumatism and obesity.
- **Abhyangam:** Special kind of oil is used to

massage the body in which strokes are given according to the condition of the patients for 45 minutes for 14 days. This treatment is for Obesity, Diabetic Gangrene, etc.

•**Nasyam:** Herbal juices and medicinal oils are applied through nose for about 30 minutes for 7 to 14 days. This treatment is usually for treating headaches, mental disorders, paralysis, and other skin diseases.

•**Snehapanam:** Medicated ghee is given internally in a proportionate increasing quantity for 8-12 days. This is useful for treating Osteo Arthritis, Leukemia, etc.

•**Kizhi:** The body is applied with herbal leaves and powder in boluses with hot medicinal oils for 45 minutes per day for 7-14 days. This treatment is for Osteo Arthritis, swellings, sports injury, etc.

•**Kativasthi:** In this treatment, Special lukewarm oil is placed over the lower back with herbal paste boundary for 45-60 minutes. It is useful for all kinds of back pains or spinal disorders.

•**Urovasthi:** Special kind of warm oil is placed over the chest for about 45 minutes. This is useful for treating asthma, heart diseases, chest pain, and other respiratory problems.

•**Ksheeradhoomam:** In this course, medicated cow milk is applied to the body or a particular part of the body. It is good for facial paralysis, speech disorders, Bell's palsy, and other facial nerve disorders.

- **Thalam:** In this process, medicated oil is mixed with a special powder and applied on the top of the head for about 20-45 minutes. This treatment is good for insomnia, migraine, ear, nose, and throat related problems.

YOGA EXERCISES AND AYURVEDA - ADJUSTING YOUR PACE OF YOGA EXERCISES AND YOGA BREATHING FOR BALANCE

When you know your Ayurvedic constitution you can make important choices regarding your speed and style of practice of yoga exercises and yoga breathing. While Yoga Exercises means a lot more than physical movement, this focus is on the physical aspect of yoga. The principles are given here can be applied both whiles in the yoga pose and day to day living to achieve comfort in the body and a quiet mind.

Let's take 3 key qualities of your body-mind according to Ayurveda: the strength of body, the temperature of the body, and stability of mind, and apply these to a yoga pose, the basic standing pose, Tadasana.

Strong Body
If you have thin bones, your constitution might be weaker than someone with a stocky build. You may both look the same holding the pose, yet

you'll begin to feel tired sooner. What's happening on the inside is different. Focus on your connection with the ground and peacefully refocus whenever the mind wanders.

Those with a stronger body can focus on yoga breathing. Yoga breathing is breathing appropriately, filling the lungs from top to bottom, or bottom to top in restful breathing. Ideally, everyone would be practicing yoga breathing while holding the pose; it's the focus of attention that is different.

Stability of Mind

If the mind is dull and lethargic, a large upward movement of the arms will stimulate the body-mind. While standing in Tadasana, raise arms overhead. You may even create a flow of movement, raising the arms on the inhalation and lowering them on the exhalation.

If on the other hand, the mind is very active, pick a spot and focus the eyes on that spot to experience some stability. You may also focus the mind on the connection of the feet with the ground. Another choice is to silently repeat a word like "strength" or "peace" on the exhalation. Choose a word that has the greatest impact on you.

Temperature of Body

Always feeling cold? Build heat with stronger

breathing during the yoga pose, especially in the cold seasons. Breathe into chest first, then abdomen second. Pay attention that your breathing is smooth and consistent. Use strong breathing to create heat in the body.

If on the other hand, your body temperature tends to be hot, avoid over-heating by breathing bottom-up, abdomen first chest second. Or you may breathe top-down smoothly, quietly and gently. Relax your effort a bit to experience more coolness and less fire.

AYURVEDIC YOGA RETREATS - A NICE EXPERIENCE WITH NATURE

Do you want to have a deep yoga experience but do not find time from your daily routine? Or you have enough time but a distraction from surrounding can't let you concentrate on your exercises and meditation? Then yoga or Ayurveda retreat is the best available solution for you. During the retreat, a family who is experienced in yoga or ayurvedic philosophy tries to make you feel all about yoga and meditation.

For this retreat, various ayurvedic and yoga centers have been established in remote areas away from the city. A day at the center can confront you with all the activities like reviving yoga, oil massage, herbal bath, relaxation, healthy nutritious meals and at the end spiritual relaxation through meditation.

A retreat center provides treatment for various diseases like nervous and muscular disorders, heart diseases, blood pressure, spondylitis, asthma, arthritis, gastritis, hair loss, etc. In an ayurvedic center an ayurvedic physician examines the patient and after proper diagnosis provides the course of treatment. Most of the treatments offered at ayurvedic centers uses originally grown seasonal vegetables and spices. These treatments are anti-aging and provide immunity to the body and mind.

Before joining any yoga or ayurvedic retreat center you have to consider certain points:

*Selection of the center:

Although all the centers are located in far places avoiding the hectic life and close to nature. But then also, you should choose the place that is farther from your place so that you can keep all the tensions home and enjoy the proximity to nature.

*Choosing program:

A no of programs is available at centers according to the illness and health of an individual. Moreover, they are available in different rates and packages. So go for a program which you can afford and which suits your health and time available to you.

Accommodation and stay:

A yoga retreat lasts for around a week and this could act as a vacation for you. So you should opt for such accommodation which is comfortable and you could spend days there feeling at home.

During any day of your yoga retreat, there are two sessions generally. One is in the morning and another one is in the evening. In the afternoon time, normal breathing exercises are being conducted as that is the time for relaxation. During the sessions of the yoga retreat, there will be no. of activities like meditation, chanting, silence, exercises, asana, etc. You should perform all such under the direction of your instructor to avoid any mishappening with you. One more thing to keep in mind is that your yoga practitioner should be an experienced man so that you can avail of the complete benefit of your program.

Besides your health, yoga or ayurvedic retreat gives you a chance to show your social aspect. There are no group activities that help you build relationships from the people over there. Such activities try to bring out another You from yourself. Keeping in mind all the above suggestions, you can make your program a life long experience for you.

CHAPTER 8: AYURVEDA AND STRESS

AYURVEDA - LEARN TO COPE WITH STRESS

Today's modern world can be a real challenge to not succumb to a host of environmental stressors. Each day our bodies are attacked by a host of microbes that work against our immune systems pulling down our overall physical health and resistance. Throughout the day more subtle emotional attacks occur as well, wearing us down, leaving us tired and having a weakened critical immune system.

Ancient people developed a treatment that puts harmony and balance back into the body and prevents the manifestation of these health issues and problems, it's called Ayurveda. It's a combination of ancient natural botanical remedies and philosophies that help you to relax, become calm, and energize mind and spirit. This practice is a path that leads you to greater personal knowledge and growth and eventually to an inner mind and body piece.

Hundreds of years before any Western culture met the rulers of India, this practice was being utilized as a form of medicine. Primarily, it was used as an aid to Indian warriors to help take away any pain they may have incurred and renewed vital energy. Over time, the practice continued to develop and expand into several different sub-specialties such as internal medicine, toxicology, and surgery. The practitioners were incredibly skilled at their tasks although they would be considered primitive when compared with modern standards.

Today Ayurveda is becoming more well known and recognized as a form of alternative medicine for people in the Western World. Some of the original texts may have been lost over time but the old wisdom and consistent principals remain in its original and authentic form. A key aspect of the medicinal system is the utilization of herbs and plant remedies, something that remains in current disciplines. Commonly known herbs such as cinnamon and cardamom have known health benefits and many treatments now involve Amalaki, the Indian fruit known for its many health benefits.

Zrii Amalaki And Ayurveda
The purity of food and drink is one of the foremost concerns in the Vedic principle. It's not enough that food should be organic but it is also preferred to harvest everything from nature when possible. Zrii Amalaki is a commonly used aid for practices that helps to soothe the human spirit and the body to become calm and relaxed. Zrii Amalaki fruit follows these principles almost exactly. The fruit is grown and harvested naturally using a technique called wildcrafting, which preserves the integrity and potency of each

fruit.

Amalaki Fruit Has Many Health Benefits

Many people have reported that Amalaki (amla - Emblica Officinalis) may aid surgery recovery and when consumed regularly help to regulate and modulate stressors. Amalaki fruit is well known for its restorative powers of regeneration and rejuvenation. Combine Vedic principles with the Amalaki fruit and you can help to transform your life.

You can feel free from many everyday common stresses and start the path towards permanent relaxation. Many Vedic principles also recommend Yoga (the sister science of Ayurveda), an offshoot of the Vedic way of life as an additional way of calming and renewing the body with gentle exercise. Even though Yoga is a type of exercise it can be as calming as most anything else.

You don't have to commit to the Ayurvedic lifestyle to obtain the health benefits of drinking the Amalaki juice. In addition to being an anti-stress agent, the fruit is an antioxidant and immunity booster. Also, most consumers of all ages report that Amalaki juice tastes good. You can take other key immunity defense superfoods and natural defense boosters and combine them with Amalaki juice to create many blended options to suit your individual needs and taste.

BEATING STRESS WITH AYURVEDIC RETREAT

The most unhealthy places on earth can be anywhere within a city. If you happen to live in a highly urbanized setting, you may have all the amenities and the conveniences within reach but you also have all the factors for catching diseases and other ailments present. It is not just the environment that can make you unhealthy though. It can probably be your way of life. Stress is an ailment that you make and the best way to beat it is to detach yourself from the very things that can make you stressful. This can be done by leaving work for a moment and take an ayurvedic retreat.

An ayurvedic retreat is not just any escape in the manner that you do with much-awaited vacation leave. It is not just rest and recreation but physical and mental rejuvenation. During the retreat, you get to have the opportunity of learning a new lifestyle, one that observes the tenets of the world's oldest form of health science, which is the Ayurveda. Although it promotes health primarily, the Ayurveda involves more, including emotional well-being and spirituality. After all, Ayurveda in the literal sense means the science of life.

For Ayurveda retreat to work effectively, a suitable environment is a major factor. If you wish to experience Ayurveda's benefits, you should not just go to a spa that is located in the heart of the bustling city you live in. The best place to do this is somewhere you can commune with nature. This is because Ayurveda is a healing process, wherein only natural remedies are applied. Some herbal supplements and oils will be used on you. All these remedies will work even better if the environment is natural too. Therefore, a garden resort will surely be advantageous towards this end. You should see to it that the location of the retreat provides you the necessary relaxing and curative atmosphere.

To achieve optimum results, you should make your Ayurveda retreat a bit longer than just a couple of days. The retreat is a brief lifestyle change, which is why two days is not enough. This is when you leave all your worries outside the place of retreat and think only of what is best for your body and mind. You will not only experience a soothing environment. You will also have massages that can remove all the acquired tension from your body. Being an alternative lifestyle, you will eat only the most healthy and yet delicious meals during your stay at a resort. A weeklong stay may be more than enough to rejuvenate you and to prepare you to experience once again the hassles of your life outside the resort.

THE BASIS FOR AYURVEDIC TREATMENT FOR STRESS

We all experience stress in our life. The problem of stress is not new. It has been plaguing mankind for generations. A surge in the number of patients who are suffering terribly due to excessive stress makes it a hot topic of discussion in the medical circle. Ayurvedic medicine for stress is truly beneficial as it focuses on solving the problem from its roots.

In Ayurvedic Treatment, it is commonly believed that there are three guns in a person, namely 'sattva' (knowledge, purity), 'rajas' (action, passion) and 'tamas' (inertia, ignorance). Eliminating stress in our day to day life is all about maintaining a balance between these three guns. To eliminate stress, it is important to have adequate sleep, eat glutton free foods, exercise daily and meditate to understand your problems.

According to Ayurveda, the problem of stress is caused when the guna of 'sattva' takes a back seat and 'rajas' or 'tamas' take over our mind and body. When the state of 'sattva' decreases, a person loses his clarity of mind, determination and ability to discriminate the right from the wrong and the other two gun's namely 'tamas' and 'rajas' takes over, which leads to stress. When a person has a high state of 'sattva', he can handle stress in a better way. He is usually calm, thoughtful and patient in his behavior towards himself and others. The opposite of this state leads to hopelessness, despair, fear, anxiety and most importantly stress.

To increase the influence of 'sattva' and reduce the negative effects of stress, take note that ayurvedic treatment for stress does not promise any short-term solution. It might take several weeks to several months to experience some changes, however, the changes would be sustainable.

Here are some Ayurvedic tips which can improve your overall life and reduce stress.

*Establish a Balance in your life

Modern existence is like living in a web of expectations from society, family and our place of work. Running after external goals can be very tiring at times. If you wish to restore your inner balance, take some time out and try to meditate in a peaceful place. The emotions which you experience during the process of meditation would tell you a lot about your mental condition. If you feel less in sync with your self, perhaps it's time for you to slow down and restore your inner balance.

*Take Adequate Rest

Taking rest always does not mean going for a long vacation. You can always delegate some not so important work to your juniors and prioritize your work schedule. Learn the art of delegation, which would help you to save some time and enjoy a short break during working hours.

• Watch What You Eat

In Ayurveda, food plays a very big role in your overall welfare. Fresh food like fruits and vegetables are said to increase the guna of 'sattva'. Any artificial or processed food like coffee, fried items, liquor or sugary products is believed to lead to an increase in 'rajas' or 'tamas'. Ayurveda strongly advocates a vegan way of life. Foods like meat or egg are said to be detrimental for the mind since they contain no life energy. Watching your diet is a great way of ensuring that you enjoy a healthy mind and body.

• Get Adequate Sleep

A lot of problem in the body is caused by sleep deprivation. Sleep deprivation can cause problems like indigestion, irritation, and fatigue which contribute to stress in a big way. Having a sound sleep without the help of drugs can cure a lot of mental problems. If you have trouble falling asleep you can try listening to light music or taking a walk post-dinner. Alternatively, you can also use aroma oil or incense sticks in your bedroom which can create a balance in your body. If these remedies don't work, you can check out some Ayurvedic herbs like Ashwagandha which can help you to rest without any side effects.

Ayurvedic remedies for stress is slow and consistent, thus aiming to cure the root of the problem. The cure lies in consciously making healthy choices concerning both lifestyle and food-related habits. Each day we make choices, and every time we choose an activity that leads to less stress, or more resilience to stress, we move toward the upward cycle of emotional balance.

CAN AYURVEDA REDUCE MEDICAL COSTS FOR CARDIOVASCULAR DISEASE, STRESS AND CHRONIC DISORDERS?

Ayurveda, the traditional health care system of India, is the world's oldest and most comprehensive system of medicine. Through the use of time-tested modalities that are natural and free of harmful side effects, Ayurveda works to prevent disease at its source, rather than working at the level of symptoms after health problems have arisen.

In 1997, the American Journal of Managed Care published an eleven-year study on Maharishi Ayurveda, a systematized revival of Ayurveda. The study used Blue Cross/Blue Shield data to analyze medical utilization patterns of individuals participating in several components of Maharishi Ayurveda, compared with matched control groups and normative data.

The study found significant reductions in medical

care utilization in those using the natural system of medicine:

• Overall medical expenditure was 63 percent lower, with 80 percent fewer hospital admissions and 55 percent fewer out-patient doctors' office visits.

• Those over the age of 45 had 88 percent fewer hospital days than the control groups.

• Analysis by disease categories showed that hospital admission rates were 92 percent lower for immune, endocrine, and metabolic disorders; 92 percent lower for cardiovascular disease; 92 percent lower for mental health and substance abuse, and 94 percent lower for musculoskeletal disorders.

Components of the Ayurveda approach to health included:

• Panchakarma treatments (traditional detoxification treatments): Research has found that these highly effective purification treatments help remove stress and impurities and stimulate the body's natural healing abilities. A customized program is designed for each person to address specific imbalances.

• Individual recommendations for diet, exercise, and optimal daily routine: Modern researchers have made great progress in understanding the molecular sequences and patterns that determine which genes get expressed. This area of study is called epigenetics. Studies show that certain "triggers"- which can range from a small exposure to toxins to various factors in one's diet, behavior or surroundings- can affect the software of our genes that determine which genes get turned on or turned off. This can affect not only the individual's body and brain for life but also the body and brain of their offspring. What these triggers are and what genes are affected differs from individual to individual. This personalized approach to health is a specialty of Ayurveda.

•Herbal preparations: Research at the Ohio State University College of Medicine indicates that certain Ayurveda herbal compounds scavenge free radicals 1,000 times more effectively that the popular anti-oxidants vitamin C and E and the much-researched Probucol (Pharmocology, Biochemistry, and Behavior, December 1992). Some researchers link free radicals with at least 80% of all diseases.

Many critics complain that medical costs today are so high because our modern health care system is a "sickness care" system. The research on Ayurveda shows that it is possible to complement modern medical approaches with effective health-promoting techniques that help prevent disease. The best way to cut the costs of health care is simply to keep people healthy. Ayurveda provides an integrated mind-body approach to restore balance within and among the various physiological systems in the body, thereby producing good physical and mental health and long vigorous life.

5 AYURVEDIC TREATMENTS FOR NATURAL STRESS REDUCTION

Stress is common and is something that most people experience. Some people suffer from professional stress, some from professional stress, and the most unfortunate ones, have both the kinds to deal with.
Stress if ignored can lead to serious health issues. Many people resort to medicines to get rid of stress. However, medicines come with side effects and should be avoided, as much as possible. So, what is the best way to treat stress?
Thanks to Ayurveda, you now can use natural remedies for stress. According to Ayurveda, simple lifestyle changes can go a long way in treating stress. There are several ayurvedic treatments for stress available and some of them include:

Lead a Healthy Lifestyle
Stress is what most people think is not only a mental thing. To get rid of stress, you need to be mentally, emotionally, and physically sound as well.
Try to wake up early in the morning - early mornings are beautiful and you would love to take a walk outside. Seeing the beauty of nature and breathing fresh air in the morning would freshen up your mind and would fill you with positivity.
You can consider doing yoga asanas,

suryanamaskara being one of them. Also, practice deep breathing.

Eat a healthy and balanced diet. You must have a smooth bowel movement.

Avoid drinking and smoking as much as possible. If you think that by drinking alcohol, you would be forgetting about the worries in your life, you are mistaken. You would indeed forget about them for something. However, once the effect of alcohol goes, everything would become normal.

You need to work towards finding a permanent solution and not a temporary one.

Opt for a Full Body Massage
Abhyanga is one great way to deal with stress. It is an Ayurvedic treatment where you need to undergo a full body massage. Lots of amounts of warm oil is used to massage on your body and this is very relaxing. If you cannot undergo a full body massage, you can at least massage your neck region, feet, and hands. This would help as well.

Try to massage your neck, hands, feet, and scalp with warm oil before going to bed every day. This would give you a good night's sleep and also reduce stress.

Meditate
Meditation is another great way to fight stress. You can consider joining meditation classes or even learn it yourself. Numerous videos are available on the Internet that helps you learn meditation.

Many studies around the world have proved that

meditation is the best way to relieve stress. It helps in reducing anxiety. It works by increasing the levels of serotonin that aids relaxation.

Herbal Remedies for Stress
According to Ayurveda, several herbs help relieve stress. Let's look at a few of them:

- **Brahmi:** Brahmi is recommended for many ailments and it has some amazing properties. Apart from helping to relieve stress, it can prevent Alzheimer's and Parkinson's disease, which have no treatment.
- **Ashwagandha:** Ashwagandha is one of the best herbs for stress and anxiety. Ashwagandha capsules are easily available and these contain the herb in its raw form. This amazing herb has anti-inflammatory properties. It helps cure various neurological disorders as well.
- **Vacha:** Having the root of his herb can reduce stress and its associated symptoms.
- **Shankhpushpi:** This herb is used to cure neurological disorders apart from relieving stress and anxiety.
- **Arjuna:** This herb has been used since time immemorial to cure many diseases. It keeps your heart healthy and also reduces stress.

Listen To Music an easy way to get relieved from stress is by listening to serene music. Music has calming effects on your nervous system and hence, helps in reducing stress. Even if you were not a music fan, listening to soothing music for a few minutes would help alleviate stress. Following a mix of these ayurvedic remedies for stress would be effective.

Ath Ayurdhamah is dedicated to restoring and maintaining the lost balance between physical, mental, emotional and spiritual health, through the understanding and practice of age-old systems of Ayurveda and Yoga. Our strength lies in understanding the body and its performance at the constitutional level and that is what we apply to our Remedies.

HEALTHY AND STRESS-FREE HEART BY AYURVEDA

According to Ayurveda literature, the heart is considered to be one of the most important "MARMA", that is, a very vital part of the human body. It is so important according to Ayurveda that it gets a separate mention in the "TRI-MARMIYA" chapter by Charaka acharya as - ASHRAYA of Atma, soul, and feelings. According to Ayurveda philosophy, how we feel in our hearts is the measure of who we are, whereas, what we think in our mind is often no more than a superficial impression, pausing momentarily through us via the senses. This way, the heart is even considered to be above mind and hence, heart diseases reflect deep-seated issues of identity, feelings, and consciousness.

Heart diseases, nowadays, are a major reason

behind death due to illness around the world. This is largely because, in today's fast and competitive life, emotions and feelings are denied and ignored. Today's life aims more towards personal achievements rather than communion with others. Many of us die of broken hearts or spiritual starvation. The saints of Ayurveda understood this fact and prescribed Satvajaya chikitsa or mental hygiene for this. Heart, according to ayurvedic philosophy, is the organ of emotions, and ayurvedic treatment for heart diseases emphasizes that emotional causes should always be considered first while treating heart ailments. Such causes include - difficulties in work or relationships, depression, low self-esteem, etc.., which usually indicate that at the inner level we are not in touch with our hearts.

According to Ayurveda, the heart is closely associated with Pranvah shrotas (Respiratory system), and Anavah shrotas (Digestive system). Ayurveda says that HRIDYA (Heart) has three functions - receiving, giving away and moving for a continuous activity to execute two earlier functions. Circulation of blood and transportation of nutrients and oxygen through it are major functions of the heart. If such a vital organ is afflicted with disease pathology, naturally all life processes are also impaired to a great extent.

Ayurveda has many herbs that are beneficial for different conditions of the cardiovascular system. Amla - The Indian Gooseberry - is considered as the best rasyan or drink which mitigates all heart ailments or hriday-dosas. This edible fruit's tissue contains protein and ascorbic acid, having concentration much higher as compared to that present in apple. Many known antioxidants, Gallic acid, Catechol, Ellagic acid, Vitamin C, carotene, and superoxide-dismutase enzyme have also been reported to be present in this fruit. As Amla is also rich in natural flavonoids, thus it promotes health vigour and stamina too, thereby reducing cholesterol and blood sugar.

Arjuna Terminalia arjuna, according to Ayurveda, is another beneficial herb. It is good for heart, cures injury inside lungs neutralizes toxins, effective in controlling fat, diabetes, and wounds and mitigates Kapha and pitta dosas. Arjuna active constituents include tannins, cardenolide, triterpenoid saponins (arjunic acid, arjunolic acid, arjungenin, arjunglycosides), flavonoids ellagic acid, calcium, magnesium, zinc, and copper. Using of Arjuna bark in milk is highly recommended for heart pain.

Today, many organizations harness the powers of these herbs and add to them the usability of the modern world by creating ayurvedic products and medicines. The products of companies like Baidyanath, Himalaya and a few others have a range of medicines that are not only easy to take but also are close to nature thereby keeping negative effects to minimal. For heart issues, there exists a range of Arjuna, Amla, and Cardiwin tonics. In Ayurveda, it is a belief that cardiac ailments, hypertension, and dyslipidemia never occur alone but are supplemented by stress, tension, and thus the herbal preparations like stress win, brain tab, ashwagandha and sarswat churan in Ayurveda aim towards not only the curing of heart issues but also act as a soothing agent for the patient, calming him from inside. This all leads to less stress along with resolving of heart ailment - leading to a long-lasting solution.

CHAPTER 9: AYURVEDA HERBS

TIPS FOR USING AYURVEDA HERBS TO CONTROL DIABETES

Diabetes is a commonly increasing disorder of the modern world and is hitting epidemic proportions. According to William Herman director of the University of Michigan's Center for Diabetes Translational Research and a consultant to the World Health Organization, diabetes is an epidemic, both in the U.S. and globally. According to recent studies, WHO estimates that nearly 350 million people worldwide have the condition.

Diabetes also is known as Diabetes Mellitus is a disorder characterized by an excess amount of blood sugar or blood glucose, and is due to the lack of the hormone insulin in the body or because the insulin present in the body is inefficient to synthesize glucose and absorb it into the body.

What is Diabetes?
Diabetes is a group of metabolic diseases in which the person suffering has a high amount of blood glucose or blood sugar, either due to inadequate insulin production in the body or because the body cells do not respond properly to

the insulin. Frequent hunger, thirst, and urination are common symptoms.

Different Types
Diabetes is of three types namely Type 1 Diabetes, An autoimmune disease; Type 2 Diabetes the body does not produce enough insulin for proper functioning and Gestational Diabetes is seen developing in women during pregnancy. Of these Type 2 is most prevalent and Type 1 least prevalent.

Common Causes
The common causes of diabetes are high blood pressure, high cholesterol, insulin deficiency or insulin resistance. It can be hereditary and also rarely due to the pancreas.

Symptoms
The main symptoms are extreme thirst, hunger, blurry vision, polyuria, weight loss, fatigue, and frequent urination.

AYURVEDA AND DIABETES

In Ayurveda diabetes is known as "Prameha". It is a chronic metabolic disorder, which makes the body unable to utilize proper use of glucose produced, resulting in hyperglycemia (high blood sugar) and glycosuria (sugar in urine). If left unattended, diabetes may lead to heart attacks, strokes, blindness, nerve damages, amputation of limbs, impotence in men and pruritus (Itching).

Ayurveda has much more scientific information on Diabetes, its symptoms, and causes and has some of the oldest records on the disease. According to Ayurveda, there are 20 forms of diabetes, 4 due to Vata dosha, 6 due to Pitta and the remaining 10 due to Kapha dosha. Diabetes is mainly a Kapha disorder.

In Ayurvedic view, Diabetes is caused mainly due to the diet increasing the Kapha dosha like sugar, rice, fats, and potatoes, lack of exercise, mental stress and strain and excessive sleep.

Diet planning, is the key factor in controlling diabetes. Proper daily exercise and restricting and reducing over-weight play another role in managing diabetes. Also, avoid smoking, sleep during daytime and stress. Practicing Yoga can help in reducing and managing stress and strain.

Ayurvedic Remedies

Some most useful Herbs for the Treatment of Diabetes are
- Bitter Gourd (Momordica charantia)
- Bael (Aegle marmelos)
- Gurmar Leaves (Gymnema sylvestrae)
- Fenugreek (Trigonella foenum graecum)
- Turmeric (Curcuma longa)
- Onion (Allium cepa)
- Nayantatra (Vinca rosa)
- Neem (Azadirachtha indica)
- Garlic (Allium sativum)
- Sagar gota (Ceasalpinia crista)

Few Ayurvedic Tips for Diabetes
•Bitter gourd is considered the best remedy for diabetes. Consume one teaspoon of bitter gourd juice daily as it reduces blood sugar levels in your blood and urine. Also having bitter gourd cooked in ghee and consuming for three months, brings down diabetes by a significant level.
•Indian gooseberry is considered to be an effective medicine for treating diabetes. A teaspoon of Indian gooseberry juice mixed with a cup of fresh bitter gourd juice, taken for two months will enable the pancreas to secrete insulin.
•Tulsi leaves are packed with antioxidants that relieve oxidative stress and have essential oils that help in lowering blood sugar levels in the body. Sugar levels can be kept under control by drinking a glass of water with 10 Tulsi (Holy Basil) leaves, 10 Neem (Azadirachtha indica) leaves and 10 Belpatras (Aegle marmelos) early morning on an empty stomach.
•Mix and grind seeds of fenugreek, turmeric, and white pepper. Have one teaspoon of this powder with a glass of milk twice daily.
•Put a cup of water into a copper vessel at night, and drink the water in the morning.
•Boil 15 fresh mango leaves in a cup of water, leave overnight, and drink the filtered water first thing in the morning, as tender mango leaves are very effective to treat diabetes by regulating insulin levels in the blood.
•Eating a healthy diet that contains vitamins and

minerals like fruits such as apples, apricots, and berries, and vegetables like carrots, beet and bitter gourd are essential for keeping your body healthy and in balancing blood sugar levels.
- Fenugreek seeds consist of fiber useful for controlling diabetes. Soak fenugreek seeds in water overnight and consume early in the morning before breakfast. The seeds can also be powdered and mixed with milk. This can enhance the secretion of glucose-dependent insulin. Repeat this remedy daily for a few months to control blood sugar levels.
- Drinking a cup of green tea on an empty stomach is found to be good for overall health. Green tea has polyphenol content, a strong antioxidant compound that helps reduce the blood sugar insulin level in the body.
- Also, recent studies have found that yogurt and curds may help lower the risk of diabetes.

Dietary Treatment

Diet planning is a key remedy for controlling diabetes. Avoid consuming sugary foods such as rice, banana, potato, cereals, and high sugar content fruits. Include bitter dishes in every meal, have leafy vegetables, black gram, soy, fish, etc.

Include vegetables like Bitter Gourd, string beans, cucumber, onion and garlic, fruits such as Indian gooseberry, Jamul fruit and grapes and grains like Bengal gram and black gram in the diet. Also consume raw vegetables and herbs as they play a key role in stimulating the pancreas and enhancing insulin production. Go for organic vegetables for better results.

To conclude diabetes is not just the lack of insulin production in the body. It is due to the poor maintenance of the body. Balancing the health of the body and the Doshas can only cure it. For this purpose, having a healthy lifestyle is significant.

9 HERBS BENEFITS IN AYURVEDA

Ayurveda tries and strives to achieve 'Fitness for all'. It originated from a Sanskrit word 'Ayu' means life and 'Veda' means knowledge. Ayurveda is supposedly created by Brahma and has a divine origin; it is considered to be a holistic science. It focuses on the entire being rather than only upon his physical health. This is one of the main benefits of Ayurveda. India's system largely depends on plant support to form a major Chunk of its medicine.

Ayurveda is the essence of old Hindu Medicare techniques, which are based on the curing the diseases from the roots. In Ayurveda, the whole body is supposed as a mutually responding system. A single part not responding well may cause a disturbance in all bodies. Ayurveda works for the aim of complete health.

The benefits of it include aging prevention, cures deep-rooted diseases, correct stress and fatigue, improves the beauty, increase life span, no more joints disorder and improves digestion. This does not have any side effects on your body, also health massage therapy is a true energizer that streamlines all your body parts. Give up all your worries!! No more tension, feel younger and confident with Ayurveda healing and therapeutic solutions.

Common Herbs used in Ayurvedic Medicines

*Amalaki (Amla or Indian Gooseberry or Emblica Officinalis)

Is the richest source of Vitamin C in its natural form. The Fresh Amla fruit contains 80% of water along with carbohydrates, fiber, protein, minerals, and vitamins. Vitamin C is an excellent antioxidant and helps to build resistance against various diseases in our body. Amalaki is one of the richest sources of powerful anti-oxidants. These anti-oxidants play a crucial role in the body to drive away free radicals and restore health. Amla is taken regularly as a dietary supplement; it counteracts the toxic effects of prolonged exposure to environmental heavy metals, such as lead, aluminum, and nickel.

*Ashwagandha (Winter Cherry or Withania Som**nifera)**

Ashwagandha is one of the main herbs for promoting ojas and rejuvenating the body in

Ayurveda. It is a well-known semen promoter and it treats impotency and infertility. Ashwagandha herb, also known as Winter Cherry is an herb that is grown in Western India and is known that may promote your overall health.

According to Ayurvedic practitioners, Ashwagandha possesses rejuvenating and life-prolonging properties. A plant with various medicinal benefits is known to assist in treating disorders like fatigue, rheumatism, impotence, premature aging and constipation.

*Arjuna (Terminalia Arjuna)

It is a cardiac tonic of high quality. Terminalia arjuna is known to be beneficial for the treatment of heart ailments since 500 BC. Terminalia Arjuna is an herb that has proven its worth in heart-related illness. No matter what kind of heart disease a person suffers from, it is given blindly in any of the heart diseases to derive benefit. Arjuna is a powerful heart stimulant, which has a sure shot effect on heart ailments.

By regular use of Arjuna, it has been seen that it provides significant cardiac protection in myocardial infarction commonly known as a heart attack.

Brahmi (Bacopa, Gotu Kola) - Brahmi is a well-known herb, worldwide used as a memory booster and mind alertness promoter. It promotes a calm, clear mind, and improves mental function. Commonly known, as Indian pennywort and Bacopa monnieri in Latin.

Since centuries Brahmi has been used as Rasayana, hence it is used to attain a long life while having energy just like a youth. It works as an antioxidant and retards aging thus keeps the person young and youthful It is also helpful in treating general body weakness and promotes energy levels like never before.

*Guggulu (Shuddha Guggulu, Guggul, Commiphora Mukul)

Commonly known as guggul in the Hindi language, is a very important and trustworthy herb in ayurvedic system of medicine.

Modern research shows that it is the prime Ayurvedic herb for treating obesity and high cholesterol. Studies show that Guggulu lowers serum cholesterol and phospholipids and that it also protects against cholesterol-induced atherosclerosis. Guggulu was seen to lower body weight in these clinical studies. Guggulu also as anti-inflammatory properties and is effective in treating arthritis and other joint pains.

*Karela (Bitter Melon, Bitter Gourd, Momordica Charantia)

Bitter melon is a valuable herb gifted to us by Mother Nature. It is also commonly known as bitter gourd, bitter cucumber, karolla, and karela. It also contains Vitamins B1, B2, B3 and C, phosphorous and fiber. Karela is one of the few

rare herbs which helps in regulating blood sugar levels in our body
It could probably reduce the patient's intake of antidiabetic drugs. Also Bitter Melon has two proteins that are thought to repress the AIDS virus.
Neem is an extraordinary blood purifier, good for al skin diseases like acne, eczema, psoriasis and teeth and gums. Neem is included in most Ayurvedic Skin products because it is as effective on an external application as through internal indigestion.
In Ayurveda, it has been safely used for over five thousand years and is a good immunity booster to prevent colds, fevers, infections and various skin diseases.

*Shilajit (Mineral Pitch, Asphaltum)

Shilajit is considered as one of the powerful anti-aging herb and rejuvenator. It is also popularly known as 'conqueror of mountains and destroyer of weaknesses'. It helps you to feel the power of growing young.
Shilajit has been used extensively in the Ayurvedic medical tradition as a treatment for a wide variety of ailments including infertility, arthritis, diabetes, cancer, depression and even schizophrenia and insanity. One of the most famous uses in India is to balance the libido and indeed many companies marketing shilajit refer to it as such!

*Triphala (Amalaki, Bibhitaki, Haritaki)

Triphala has got the properties of three famous nutrients: amla, haritaki, and bibhitaki. The advantage of this formula is that it is milder in action and more balanced than any of the three alone. These three fruits are Amalaki, Haritaki, and Bibhitaki. These fruits have been used for ages in ayurvedic natural remedies. They complement each other in such a way as to provide significant benefits to our health.

Triphala is vastly considered as one of the most important medicines Ayurveda has ever provided to the world. The uses for which Triphala is today internationally acclaimed like for Digestive Problems, Flatulence, Gout Care, Liver Disorders, Nervous Disorders, Obesity, Ocular Problems & many more.

*Tulsi (Holy Basil, Ocimum Sanctum)

Known as the queen of herbs, Holy Basil is renowned for its spiritual and religious significance and has at the same time carved a niche for itself in the traditional Indian system of medicine.

Holy basil is also a major ingredient of many Ayurvedic cough syrups. it is a good stress reliever, Immunity enhancer, Nervine debility, Fever, Sore throat, disorder, Kidney stones, Heart problems, Tensions and stress, Oral infection, Eyes related problems and modern research has found it to be good for Respiratory problems, Cold, Fever and all types of a Cough.

Eventually, it was introduced in our lives and slowly but surely it gained momentum with time. Ayurveda practices include various therapeutic measures for an understanding of life.

LEARNING, TEACHING AND PRACTICING AYURVEDA

Living life healthy isn't always easy, but the rewards are priceless. Practicing Ayurveda in your life can produce benefits you've never dreamt of. These benefits are not just those associated with your body's health. These benefits can transform your entire life into a state of being that is not only peaceful but stress-free and stronger. When we think of stronger, the image of a bodybuilder may come in the picture, but when the word strong is put in the same context as Ayurveda, it means strength in health.

The look of peak health isn't large muscles and lifting weights, even if society looks at it this way. Peak health is being in tune with one's mind body and soul. This can be attained through the practice of Ayurveda. Many people aren't aware of Ayurveda and the benefits one gets while living in tune with your self. This means knowing how your body works and what it takes to strive for complete health. Complete health doesn't just mean eating right and watching calories. Complete health is Ayurveda.

Many people have come to know the concept of living the Ayurveda lifestyle. With this comes much learning for the students of Ayurveda. Once a student masters the practices, they often become the teacher spreading the ancient teachings of this 5000-year-old Indian medicine. Although it began in India, it has spread to many parts of the world.

With a simple search, you can find individuals who are willing to teach this method of living as well as groups. But the amazing thing is you will now find schools that will provide you with the entire teachings of Ayurveda, either online or in the classroom.

With all the stresses that the world today can dump on us, we fre*q*uently search for ways to relieve the daily stress. Some look to Doctors, others seek medication or alcohol. With Ayurveda, all these vises can be eliminated and once mastered; the thought of stress will not even be an issue. Your life will be transformed and your mind will be in tune with your body and what is needed to keep it healthy and happy for many years to come. It is said that Ayurveda is the fountain of youth.

So whether you are looking to learn to live longer, happier and healthier, or looking to cure what ails you, or possibly master this ancient holistic healing method to teach others how to live in harmony with Ayurveda, just remember it takes a lot of discipline, determination, and dedication. It will not happen overnight and it's not a simple formula for healing when you are sick. Although some of the methods can be applied for those who just seek a holistic approach in times of need, for the full benefits, a complete transformation into a lifestyle of Ayurveda will bring you long and happy days for many years to come.

MEDITATION AND AYURVEDIC HEALING

Ayurvedic healing employs many methods of treatment, concentrating on treating the person as a whole instead of the physical body alone. Among color and gem therapies, herbal medicines and yoga, meditation as therapy is the one that seems to conflict most with western medicine.
Why? One fundamental reason is the different perspectives on healing. A conventional medical doctor primarily will treat physical symptoms and attempt to target a physical malfunction as the origin of the disease. Nearly always, this is done through pharmaceutical medications.
On the other hand, an Ayurvedic doctor will treat a patient based on a long list of individual criteria that includes lifestyle and emotional evaluations,

as well as physical. Based on the belief that poor health is a result of some imbalance somewhere in life, the Ayurvedic professional will try to determine what area is out of balance and then go about correcting it through traditional treatments of Ayurvedic healing. Meditation is a part of every therapeutic regimen because it is how the mind can make its contribution to the healing process.

The role of meditation in the Ayurvedic healing is to enlist the patient's mental and spiritual faculties to aid in restoring balance to the bodily system. Through meditation, the patient can be relieved of the stress and anxiety that often accompany illness. It also can improve the quality of sleep and enhance the patient's self-esteem. It replenishes and restores energy levels.

Using meditation as part of the overall treatment plan also has its physical benefits. The practice has proven to be effective in reducing stress levels and blood pressure. Additionally, it lowers the respiration and heart rates while increasing the flow of blood. Ayurvedic healing is about restoring harmony and balance in a patient's life. Meditation works to provide the emotional and spiritual muscle needed to assist the physical body in reclaiming that balance.

AYURVEDA - 7 DISTINCTIVE DIFFERENCES BETWEEN MODERN AND AYURVEDIC MEDICINES

The medical systems, whether it is Ayurveda or the conventional Allopathic, Modern, medicines, each has its advantages and disadvantages. Without any intention to criticize any system of medicines and/or to force you to follow a certain medical practice, the article presents a detailed comparison between modern and Ayurvedic medicines.

Approach

Modern medicines treat the physical body, considering each organ or component as separate from the other. Thus, we find specialists in modern medicines. For instance, a cardiologist will most likely refer you to a gastrologist if you came to him complaining of suffering from severe hurt burn

In contrast, the field of Ayurveda holistically treats the whole body. This system believes that a complete Ayurvedic physician is one who is conversant with all systems of medicines associated with Ayurveda. To the Ayurvedic practitioner, body mind and spirit are connected and treating any condition involves balancing all three aspects.

•Side Effects

It is a common fact that modern medicines are full of side effects. For instance, a woman taking birth control pills often finds herself getting obese.

In contrast, Ayurveda is based on herbs, which are found in nature and Ayurvedic natural herbal remedies do not have any side effects.

•Natural Treatment

In the last few decades, the influx of Ayurvedic knowledge in the west has sensitized them to the concept of natural treatment but they are far away from applying the understanding of natural medicines. Conventional medicines believe in prescribing synthetic and chemical substances to treat any condition

In contrast, Ayurveda believes in herbalism, which is derived from nature. They believe that intimate communion with nature is the only way to gain ideal wellness.

•Evidence-Based

Conventional medicine is purely evidence-based even though modern doctors engage in lots of trial and error. How many times have you visited a doctor who gave you a particular medicine for an ailment only to be changed on your next visit?

In contrast, it is a misconception that Ayurveda is not based on scientific principles. Ayurveda has its own set of principles which is followed by every Ayurvedic practitioner religiously. Ayurvedic treatment is nature-based and the system follows the natural wisdom and universal truth that plants and the derived herbal remedies can be used to prevent and, if necessary, to cure all health issues. It has been said that "there is no beginning and there is no end to Ayurveda." Its range of knowledge cannot be contained in books.

---

*Roots

Modern medicines and treatment are more inclined towards suppressing the symptoms of a disease rather than eradicating it from its root. A simple case - when you visit a doctor when you have flu, often the doctor prescribes medicines that will suppress the symptoms. But does the medicine cure it? No.

In contrast, Ayurvedic remedies are not concerned with suppressing symptoms. Initially, the prescribed remedies will, very often, intensify the symptoms so that the problem can be treated from its root. Rather than suppress a fever, the Ayurvedic doctor will allow it to rise, while controlling it, to allow the high fever to destroy whatever bacteria that has invaded the organism.

*Diet and Lifestyle

Modern medicine rarely considers the diet and lifestyle of the suffering person. They are just interested in the disease and in doing so disease is never prevented and, at best, it is suppressed until the next episode. However, in the last few years, modern medicine practitioners have slowly warmed up to the idea of including the diet and lifestyle too while prescribing treatment.

In contrast, Ayurveda believes that our well-being depends on what we eat and the way we manage our life. A healthy diet, a balanced lifestyle that includes spiritual enhancement, will ensure balance and harmony in the life of a person. If this balance is maintained, there is no need for any kind of medicines. It is only when the balance is disrupted that health problems arise.

*Detoxification

Modern medicine is more concerned with suppressing the symptoms, as mentioned above. It simply does not understand the concept of prevention through body detoxification, for example. Even if a handful of doctors are aware, they shy away from recommending it because it is not prescribed under the rules of modern medicine.

In contrast, detoxification is the basis of all Ayurvedic remedies. They stress the fact that removing the toxins from the body plays the most important role in eradicating the disease-causing factors that will also prevent the disease from erupting again and again.

These are the 7 primary differences between Ayurveda and Modern, conventional, medicine. They are brought to you with the hope that they will invoke in you the curiosity and hunger to explore and discover for yourself the enormous benefits that Ayurveda has to offer.

YOUR HEALTH AND AYURVEDA - SEE THE BIG PICTURE, DON'T GET STUCK IN DETAILS

These days with so much information available about every diet, every individual food, every additive and every form of exercise, it's easy to become obsessed and end up a victim of information overload. To how do you separate the useful information from the irrelevant and find a path that resonates with what you need?

Also, very often information from respected sources seems to conflict with information from other respected sources, which makes it even harder to decide what's valuable to you. So what's going on?

Well, all expert writers will be writing from their particular standpoint, their sphere of learning, and their particular body type and imbalances, (whether present or past), however hard they try to cater to the needs of others. There's nothing wrong with this; it's just how it happens, and it doesn't make any of these experts any less, well, an expert in their fields...

However, it's up to us to find our unique body types so we can sift through the information and find what we need at any given time. One expert's knowledge might be exactly what you need at the moment, but don't just discard the writings of another who you might not completely agree with, because this time next year, with a different set of physical imbalances, and a move to a hotter country (for example), what they had to say might be just what you need.

This is where the ancient Indian science of Ayurveda comes in. The superb classification system that Ayurveda runs on - the three 'doshas', Vata, pitta, and Kapha - covers absolutely everything in creation. Once certain simple principles are learned, it's easy to see whether food, or an exercise, or a seasonal change, or even your preferred bedtime, falls under one of these doshas.

If you have an imbalance of Vata dosha, which might perhaps manifest as restlessness, weight loss, headaches, poor sleeping patterns, etc, you can easily turn your attention to the things that balance Vata - routine, good sound sleep, warm nourishing food, gentle exercise, meditation, and fewer stimulants and TV.

If you have a Kapha imbalance, perhaps showing up as sluggishness, weight gain, sinus, and allergy problems, etc, you can choose foods and activities that reduce Kapha, such as more salads, vigorous exercise, getting up early, etc, etc.

So, what Ayurveda does is help you to gain more intuition about your health by generally simplifying things down to just three key choices. Once you understand these principles, you can reduce the whole chaotic search for the next ideal diet or lifestyle down to whether it supports the balancing of the dosha that you need to balance at the time.

Simple!

For example, you are trying to decide whether

you need to follow a low-carb diet full of raw veggies and salads, or to follow a more regular diet, just watching calories and making sure the ingredients are wholesome. Which do you choose?

Well, I don't know, because I'm not you!

YOU are the one who can answer that when you know exactly what you are trying to achieve in the context of the Ayurvedic system, and then it all becomes clear.

Of course, the ultimate goal is just to pick and choose foods and activities that are best for you purely from your intuition, which when developed is the most accurate way to stay on the right path. But for the moment, while you are developing that intuition, don't get distracted and bogged down in details about the effects of that tiny amount of one 'E' number on your packet of soup, or the exact effect that pasteurized and homogenized milk has on the endocrine system. Let Ayurvedic principles help you to see the big picture and keep your sanity... and in the long run, your health!

CHAPTER 10: AYURVEDA SOLUTION FOR BETTER SLEEP

AYURVEDIC SOLUTIONS FOR BETTER SLEEP

Ayurveda is a form of alternative medicines that were used in the Indian subcontinent during the Vedic and the Aryan civilization. The word is a combination of two similar words, which, after splitting up means ayus meaning life and Veda meaning knowledge and roughly it sums up to the science of life. The whole subject of Ayurveda deals with measures of healthy living, along with therapeutic measures that relate to physical, mental, social and spiritual harmony. It is remarkable to state that Ayurveda is one of the very few traditional and primitive systems of medicines that involves surgery. In the system of Ayurveda, the teacher or the guru gave a solemn address and he directs the students to a life of chastity, honesty, and vegetarianism.

Ayurvedic Methods for Better Sleep
The goal of an Ayurvedic approach for better sleep is to create more ojas, the finest product of digestion that provides energy, enthusiasm, happiness, clarity of thinking, better coordination between the heart and mind, and immunity.

Researches have concluded that only the deepest, most restful sleep, called Stage Four sleep creates Ojas. Good quality of sleep is very much essential as it provides deeper rest to the mind and senses, and enhances
the capacity for mental and physical work the next day. From the Ayurvedic point of view, there are three basic types of sleeping disorders. The first one is caused by Vata imbalance or mental stress.

Sufferers may toss and turn, unable to fall asleep because their mind is whirling. This may be overcome by eating more sweet, sour, and salty foods and three cooked meals at the same time every day. It also recommends the intake of herbal green tea before going to bed. The second disorder is caused by Pitta imbalance or emotional trauma. In this one may fall asleep fine but wake up every 90 minutes with heart racing, muscles tense, and emotions of fear, anger, and sadness. The third one is due to the Kapha imbalance that can result in long hours of sleep and waking up unrefreshed.

A common recommendation for these disorders includes avoiding spicy foods, eating sweeter, bitter, and astringent tastes, avoid skipping meals eating enough dinner so one doesn't wake up hungry.

SUKHANIDRA - BETTER SLEEP WITH AYURVEDA

Sukhanidra is a form of Ayurvedic treatment aimed at pacifying the mind and to treat such conditions like insomnia (sleep deprivation), anxiety and depression.

Sukhanidra (sukanidra) means calm sleep or sound asleep.

Insomnia or lack of sleep is, in fact, a serious problem that can cause other disorders like anxiety and depression. A good night's sleep can reduce anxiety and depression.

Sukhanidra treatment program is aimed at creating a pacifying environment to facilitate sleep. The treatments include body and head massage with medicated oils. Sirovasty, thalam, kshetra Dhara, thaila Dhara, etc are employed.

The person is also given medicines to strengthen the immune system and blood circulation. Yoga and meditation further pacify the soul of the person. He or she will be able to sleep calmly at night, effectively reducing anxiety and stress-related problems.

Sukhanidra (also spelled sukanidra, sukha nidra, suka nidra) treatment lasts for 7 to 21 days, during which the person is kept in a pacifying environment. The person receives full-body medicated oil massage, head massage with medicated oil and spends time doing yoga and practicing meditation techniques.

A person can expect immediate positive results in the form of reduced stress, increased confidence, better immune system, and calm sleep.

Nidra in Malayalam means sleep. This is a treatment aimed at ensuring calm, sound sleep to pacify troubled minds and souls. Though it appears to be a very simple treatment, the benefits are manifold. Seasoned Ayurveda practitioners in Kerala give good treatment for people from parts of Kerala, India and around the world.

SLEEP THERAPY - 10 BENEFITS OF AYURVEDA

By providing ways about diet and a person's lifestyle, Ayurveda aims at retaining the health of the people and improving the health of the ailing. It also provides a harmonious existence among the three components that constitute a human being-mind, body, and soul, it is believed that lifestyle and diet can make this possible. The following procedure on a chosen diet can have immeasurably benefit to the whole being of a person.

*Lemon juice

Squeezing a half a lemon in a cup of hot water

and taking it before breakfast is vastly beneficial to your health. Benefits accrued from taking lemon juice include improving digestion, fights bacteria, boosts appetite and cleans ones' digestive tract.

•Having all your senses with you during meals time

It's often the case that eating has become a mechanical process that simply involves shoveling food into your mouth without tasting or even smelling it. Attune all your five senses to the meal you are taking from smelling the sweet aroma to tasting the succulent delicacies. The enthusiastic reception of a meal triggers other biological functions like tickling salivary glands and readying the digestive system. This is important in Ayurveda.

•Having frequent lunches

In Ayurveda, Missing lunch is a dietary crime equal to none. Digestion and subsequent absorption are at their peak during this time and food eaten at this time is most beneficial to you. Avoid missing lunches for better health.

•Light meals before going to bed

Night accords your body space to regain its energy and gives time to the digestive system to work on the food you had eaten during the day. Heavy eating at night overloads your digestive system and makes it difficult for food eaten to be absorbed and assimilated.

•Rest after eating

In the world clogged with countless activities, it might seem a bad idea to take a breather after eating. In Ayurveda, resting after a meal is synonymous with sound health. That rest encourages a body to efficiently digest the food taken before the setting in of metabolism.

•Keeping yourself well hydrated

Drinking water is a prerequisite for a healthy body. It assists in digestion and absorption of food nutrients. It also a key tool in excretion where the harmful elements are removed. Above all, water offers vital help in the melting down of fat.

•Drink lukewarm water laced with aromatic herbs

Lukewarm water assists in the smooth passage of food through the digestive tract and provokes the digestive enzymes into action. The aroma from the herbs is an olfactory stimulant that tickles the taste buds and gets a palate ready to enjoy a meal.

*Meals unaccompanied by ice-drinks

This is a cardinal rule in this therapy. Very low temperatures inhibit digestive enzymes rendering the digestion process slower. Instead, take warm water or milk.

*Leaving the day's work at the office

It's always the case that people carry office work at home and in so doing, they violate the tranquil and serene home climate by turning their homes into an office. Don't carry any assignments that will strain on you at your home.

*Deep meditation before sleeping

Ayurveda's key aim is to create a harmonious and balanced existence between the mind, the soul and the body. Meditating before sleep brings closer these three components and improves on the holistic development of a person.

As much as it will be possible, follow the instructions above and win the benefits. As you can see, they are all cost-free.

HOW TO CURE INSOMNIA THROUGH AYURVEDA?

Insomniacs commonly complain that they are unable to get to sleep at night due to unwanted thoughts, worries, and concerns. Nearly half of all insomnia cases are due to emotional issues such as stress, anxiety, and depression.

According to Ayurveda the amount of sleep you need depends on your body type. Vata body type can manage with six to seven hours of sleep. Imbalance of veta causes insomnia.

The brain works best at night according to experts. However, thoughts, worries, and fears that are usually inhibited during the day surface at bedtime. If you try to stop them forcefully, they will grow stronger, because you will be giving them more attention. To reduce the *q*uantity and strength, you have to learn to ignore them.

- Apply ksheerabala thailam on the scalp, ears, and soles before a shower.
- Spend at least 20 to 30 minutes every day practicing yoga. You could also make it a habit of spending a few minutes in meditation every day.
- Instead of relying on your mind to help you rem0ember all the tasks that you need to do the next day, write them down so you will not end up worrying about forgetting them.
- A warm bath before sleep before bedtime can help prepare you for sleep.
- Don't drink caffeinated beverages in an hour before bedtime.

- Take a teaspoon of ashwagandha (Withania somnifera) with warm milk at bedtime
- Keep your bedtime and wake time consistent. However, the less you know what time it is, the better you'll sleep; hide clocks, if any, in your bedroom.
- Improve your sleeping environment in any way you can, for example, keep it dark and soundproof, and wear earplugs if you think sounds are preventing you from falling asleep.
- For about a minute, let thoughts come freely into your mind. Try to look at them with a lack of interest as if watching a boring movie. An ignored thought ultimately goes away.
- Practice Savasana: lie down straight on a mat. Beginning from your toes, start paying attention to every muscle in your body. Work your way upright to your head. If you feel any muscle is tense, attempt to relax it be following it to limp.

FIND BENEFICIAL & NATURAL REMEDIES FOR INSOMNIA THROUGH AYURVEDA

Insomnia is also known as 'Indra' in Ayurveda. According to Ayurvedic scholars, the 'pitha' and the 'doshas' are the main reasons for giving you sleepless nights. It is a deprived condition wherein a person doesn't have proper rest and sleep, which affects his entire health and daily functioning.

Some prime causes of insomnia are a busy lifestyle, high work stress, irregular sleeping cycles, addiction to cell phones, and other kinds of modern devices. Restful sleep, a balanced diet, and a simple lifestyle are the three main foundations of any Ayurvedic treatment.

The wealth of Ayurvedic herbs and different types of medicines for Anidra or insomnia:

•**Brahmi Herb:** This herb is a power-packed tonic for the human brain, which helps in improving your mental health. Brahmi is also an effective tranquilizer and a wonderful Ayurvedic medicine for insomnia. Just taking Brahmi powder or Brahmi tea before going to bed can induce a deep slumber.

•**Ashwagandha Herb:** It is used as an Ayurvedic tonic for providing vigor and energy. It helps in coordinating the reflexes of your brain and mind. And it results in getting good quality sleep. The normal Ayurvedic treatment for insomnia with Ashwagandha herb is usually an herbal powder. The dosage can be taken along with a glass of warm milk.

•**Valerian Herb:** The Indian herb valerian helps to clear out body toxins, especially from the colon, joints, blood vessels, and nerve channels. This flushing activity rejuvenates and infuses new vitality in the body. However, valerian herb should be taken in combination with other herbal concoctions.

•**Vacha Herb:** This herb is used to treat common ailments such as headache, cold and insomnia. Vacha is known as 'Acorus Calamus' and is an effective Ayurvedic medicine. In India, the herb is rubbed against a stone and the paste is given to tiny tots for improving their speech and memory.

There are numerous Ayurvedic herbal remedies for insomnia. Other medicines include Nidrodaya rasa, pipplimula churna, vatakulantaka, and swamamakhshik bhasma. They may be available in powder or churna form at ayurvedic health stores.

According to Ayurvedic studies, primary root causes of sleeplessness are as follows:

- Toxins accumulated in the body that blocks natural circulation
- Poor dietary habits and low nutrition levels
- An imbalanced nervous system and a weak digestive system
- Constant accumulation of mental stress coupled with the tired physical condition
- Low natural immunity power
- Total disturbance of the natural biological clock

The allopathic drugs often ignore these root causes and provide medications for a temporary cure. Many of the body factors are not addressed and as a result, the condition soon becomes chronic. Innumerable people suffer from insomnia and try to find transitory or short-term relief.

However, Ayurveda delves deep into the intricate workings of the human mind and body. It prepares you to transform and achieve perfect health through gradual lifestyle changes. A reputed Ayurvedic practitioner may advise you to take up yoga and other breathing exercises to balance the doshas in your body. Correct yogic practices can build your natural immunity against diseases and bring about the perfect balance of the bodily elements. Once the balance is restored, the insomnia condition is automatically rectified.

ANCIENT AYURVEDA SCIENCE AND INSOMNIA

Since ancient times, before the advent of conventional allopathy doctors, the great science of Ayurveda was used for healing mind and body illnesses. Ayurvedic medicines are like a vast ocean offering 100% natural herbal medications.
Ayurveda is part and parcel of Indian heritage. The expert Ayurvedic physicians believe that olden science is based on three basic principles mainly; perception interference and oral testimony. These experts use their knowledge and experience to treat insomniac patients, who lose sleep regularly. They emphasize the importance of timely sleeping habits and waking up early. A good night's sleep can refresh you and clear your mind of all negative vibrations. Similarly, getting undisturbed sleep at night is very important to relax the brain as well as mind and for the flow of peaceful thought patterns.

Ath Ayurdhamah is dedicated to restoring and maintaining the lost balance between physical, mental, emotional and spiritual health, through the understanding and practice of age-old systems of Ayurveda and Yoga. Our strength lies in understanding the body and its performance at the constitutional level and that is what we apply to our Remedies.

Ayurveda is an ancient traditional medicine mainly found in India and other nearby countries. It refers to knowledge of long life and believes in the maintenance of equal life forces to achieve long and healthy life.

AYURVEDIC PRINCIPLES

Ayurvedic principles dwell on maintaining balance and harmony within your body. Your whole system forms a constitution called Prakriti. Ayurvedic practitioners believe that your body is made of five primary elements including air, water, ether, fire, and earth. Every individual possesses a unique characteristic of life forces or dosas.

There are three life forces or energies to maintain and sustain as you go along your life such as:
- Vata dosas
- Pitta dosas
- Kapha dosas

Inequalities in doas in our body can lead to

malfunction and disease. Accumulation of excessive amounts of any dosas suggests a dietary and lifestyle changes to equalize the life forces. In case of toxicity, cleansing or also known as Pancha Karma is necessary to remove the toxin out of your system.

Ayurvedic practitioners base their diagnosis and treatment on the imbalances of three life forces. They will diagnose a patient using their five senses to assess the physical and mental manifestation of any imbalances.

Applying Ayurvedic Principles

Ayurvedic medicine emphasizes the significance of balance and harmony to maintain vitality. Suppression of your natural urges can lead to any disease but the fulfillment of urges should be kept at a moderate level. Ayurvedic Medicine utilizes a wide array of herbal medicines, specialized diet, massage, exercise and meditation to maintain balance. They believe that suppression of any disease is possible through the help of the environment rather than conventional ways like surgery, powerful drugs, and stem cell.

Furthermore, Ayurveda views sleeplessness and anxiety as a problem in the Vata doas. Nevertheless, some studies suggest that some imbalances in Pitta doas and Kapha doas can be health challenges that lead to the manifestation of sleeping disorders and anxiety. Ayurveda believes that the following conditions might be the cause of insomnia:

- Presence of toxins in the blood
- Poor dietary intake
- Slow or fast digestion
- Imbalance in the nervous system
- Presence of stress and anxiety
- Altered immune function and resistance to disease
- Disturbed biological sleep rhythm

Some of this manifestation includes the upset stomach, respiratory problems, asthma, hormonal imbalance, and slow metabolism. These health conditions may alter your day to day functioning and sleeping cycle that in turn contribute to your sleep deprivation or insomnia.

Ayurveda helps every individual to cope with stress, sleep deprivation and anxiety through the help of herbal remedies like:

- Ashwagandha
- Jatamansi
- Brahmi
- Celery
- Passionflower

Safety and potency is a concern with Ayurvedic medicine. Some studies suggest that herbs containing powerful components may lead to toxicity. As with any medicine or drug, misuse and overdosage can be a big problem in Ayurvedic medicine. The safest solution is to consult everything with your Ayurvedic practitioner regarding health issues, dosage, and interactions of various remedies.

Other alternative Ayurvedic medicine includes exercise and meditation such as yoga and deep breathing. Meditation and exercise are usually a safe method to balance your physical, mental and spiritual state. Ayurveda believes that there is a connection between your body, mind, and soul. Regular use of meditation in your daily activities can enhance a sleep rhythm that will enable you to have a good sleep. It will eliminate daily stress, anxiety, and worry that might be the cause of your sleeplessness.

An Ayurvedic specialized diet will help you to select foods that will favor your condition. Foods that are easy to digest, full of nourishment, cleanse your blood and strengthen your immunity against disease.

Hence, Ayurveda believes in your body's inner natural capacity to heal your sleep disorders. It is your natural response to any disease in a given situation. This holistic approach can be your edge against the manipulation and toxicity of conventional medicine for health prevention and restoration. It is an alternative way to combat your insomnia naturally and effectively.

AYURVEDA: A PERFECT CURE FOR NIGHT DISCHARGE TREATMENT

The Ayurvedic medicines harbor treatment for various diseases. These medicines are also very effective in treating various sexual deficiencies in men. The Nocturnal emission or nightfall is a nightmare for various men. In this, the men ejaculate involuntarily during sleep due to dreams or because of the hormones.

The Ayurveda harbors treatment for this disease. There are various species of plants that help in providing strength to the reproductive system. Using these plants and herbs, the treatment for nigh fall is possible. Various sexologist specialists are offering this treatment. They are using naturally occurring substances to offer a cure for this disease.

First of all, let me discuss what exactly happens in this disease. In this disease, the oozing of semen takes place unintentionally. This activity adversely affects the health of the male. The emission of this results in a very dangerous disease popularly known as premature ejaculation. In this, the male ejaculates prematurely during sexual intercourse. This eventually results in dissatisfaction between the partners.

The treatment for night discharge is possible. Though there are several medicines available in the market, yet herbal drugs are considered as the best remedy for this disease. In this, the main ingredients of the medicines are roots, stems, and leaves of the plants. In this, other ingredients like vitamin supplements, minerals, and various other naturally occurring substances are also used to make these medicines more effective.

The working principle of these medicines is very simple. These minerals and vitamins rich medicines help in improving the blood circulation through the body tissues. The medicines improve blood circulation in the reproductive system. This eventually results in providing nourishment and strength to the muscles of the penis. These medicines improve the strength of the muscles which results in curing the night discharge.

Several advantages are associated with these medicines. Unlike other medicines, these don't contain any harmful chemicals. Owing to this these medicines don't offer any side effects. These medicines are developed from naturally occurring substances and don't offer any side effects. Another advantage associated with these medicines is that their medicines don't develop any wild behavior. Apart from this, these medicines offer results promptly. One can easily get a perfect cure for this disease promptly while consuming these drugs.

Several doctors are offering night discharge treatment. They are offering treatment that is based on these herbal medicines. Apart from this, certain precautionary measures help in curing this disease. Some of the measures are discussed here that help in offering perfect health standards.

One has to perform exercises daily to get a cure for this disease. In addition to this, for timely delivery, it is recommended to take the curd in the diet. This helps in improving the strength of the reproductive system.

Certain activities are also important during the cure. One should not indulge in reading sexual or pornographic content. Apart from this, one should also not indulge in watching porn related content or videos.

These activities also affect the simulation of the reproductive organ. Thus, the simulation increases the production of the semen, which eventually results in the release or the discharge. So, one must prevent itself from watching porn-related literature and videos.

If you follow the above-mentioned advice, then it will help you in getting a cure from the night discharge. If someone is suffering from this disease, then he should choose a treatment based on herbal medicines. These medicines will help you in getting better health.

CONCLUSION

Ayurveda is composed of two words: ayur meaning life, and Veda meaning knowledge. So you can think of Ayurveda as the "knowledge of life" or the "science of life". The main emphasis of Ayurveda is on the prevention of diseases. And that is where it differs from modern medicine, where the emphasis is on treating diseases.

Ayurveda also puts a lot of emphasis on the rejuvenation of our body and increasing our life span. And the purpose of increasing the life span is so that it gives us more time to do good deeds, share the wisdom that comes or ideally should come with age, and leave the world a better place than we inherited, and not exactly for having wild sex at age 70. Not that there's anything wrong with it, but I don't think that's what the rishis visualized.

www.ingramcontent.com/pod-product-compliance
Lightning Source LLC
Chambersburg PA
CBHW052357220526
45465CB00003BB/1132